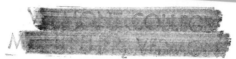

CHILDREN OF MENTALLY ILL PARENTS
Problems in Child Care

COMMUNITY MENTAL HEALTH SERIES
SHELDON R. ROEN, EDITOR

CHILDREN OF MENTALLY ILL PARENTS
Problems in Child Care

Elizabeth P. Rice
Associate Professor of Social Work in Public Health, Emerita

Miriam C. Ekdahl
Assistant in Social Work

Leo Miller
Formerly Research Associate in Social Work

*all of the Department of Maternal and Child Health,
Harvard School of Public Health, Boston, Massachusetts*

Behavioral Publications   New York

Library of Congress Catalog Card Number 71-140046
Standard Book Number 87705-018-X
Copyright © 1971 by Behavioral Publications

BEHAVIORAL PUBLICATIONS, 2852 Broadway–Morningside Heights,
New York, New York 10025

Printed in the United States of America

Contents

Foreword

Some years ago we were asked if we could say whether the children of mentally ill parents in Massachusetts were receiving the child health care and other kinds of care required for their basic needs. We did not know and, so far as our examination of the literature went, not a great deal could be learned from other studies. It seemed important to us to learn something about the extent to which families were able to assure continued satisfaction of their children's basic needs when one of the parents was mentally ill. We wanted to know something about the ability of families in such situations to manage from their own resources, and the extent to which community resources were called upon for help or found ways of initiating a helping relationship.

We were, of course, aware of the limitations of services provided for children *after* deprivation or neglect had already resulted in impairment of health or disorders of behavior or of emotional development. The need to identify *situations* in the social environment in which there exists an increased risk of such impairment was clear. Primary prevention can become available most efficiently (and perhaps only) if such situations of heightened risk are identified so that the families needing evaluation, and potentially help, can be readily reached and brought within an articulated network of health and social services.

Children of mentally ill parents form one group, not negligible in number, in which we thought there was likely to be an increased risk of insufficient or inappropriate care of children. Families with a mentally ill parent with children at home are not always easily identified. In many instances, however, they do pass through portals of entry into community institutions or agencies and, once identified, staff members should be able to initiate action to minimize the chances that the

vii

children would be exposed to unnecessary hazards. Two such portals were selected in these studies: the mental hospital and the emergency service of the general hospital. Still other portals that might be utilized with advantage are suggested by the authors.

Having found the ways to locate families with a mentally ill parent, the next question is whether skilled assessment of the situation can be arranged, and whether the plan of care indicated by the assessment can, in fact, become available. "Available" in this context does not mean "ultimately" at the end of a long waiting list. It means immediately available. When the development of young children is the issue, timeliness is the element without which much may be lost. It is a question, in many cases, of *now* or *never mind*. The findings of these studies are not brightly cheerful reading as to the adequacy, effectiveness, and timeliness of existing services.

Severe mental illness in a parent under certain circumstances creates problems for the children for which there is no single reasonably satisfactory solution. The arrangements for their health and well-being and rearrangements in a given family situation, the services offered, and the long-term solution which is to be worked for, are all, at present, matters of judgment, based upon knowledge and experience. At the present time, as the authors of these studies have shown, in too many instances there is no one to accept the delicate responsibility of making the necessary judgments, with the result that the children are left to vicissitudes under generally unplanned arrangements worked out without counsel or assistance by parents, relatives, or friends. What happens to the children in such a situation becomes largely a matter of chance.

As Younghusband (1964) wrote:

We human beings know little enough about ourselves, individually and as members of society, in all conscience, but we do know a good deal more than we practice, and we could add to the knowledge we have more rapidly if we used it and reflected upon the results. It is profoundly unethical if in dealing with people we employ methods that are less skilled, less intelligently compassionate, than they need be. If we use hit-or-miss methods to a greater extent than we must, then we will miss more often than we need, and in so doing damage or fail to help others more often than is inevitable.

In this series of studies, two methods were designed and tested in practice in an effort to create a framework for direct social service for the families by means of which effective channels could be set up to available community child health and other child care services. Comparison with control groups provided the experience that forms the basis for proposals for next steps in organization of community services so that they can become more responsive to the needs of families such as these.

These studies are probes into an aspect of child health in which illness of a parent, the social environment of the child, and the child's health and development influence each other. Severe illness of a parent—above all of a mother—poses a potential threat to the integrity of the family. One can see from these studies how far we have to go not only to achieve comprehensive health care for the individual (the parent), but even more, to make it a part of inclusive care for the family. Until a national health program can provide inclusive health care for all families, the minimum goal ought to be inclusive care for mothers and their children, and, if the lessons of these studies are to be applied, high priority is needed for those families threatened with loss or disability of the mother.

The difficulty is that when psychiatric care (and medical care in general) is given to the parent, it almost always takes place in a framework which does not assure a system of care and preventive services for the children. This fault cannot be corrected solely by increasing the quantity of psychiatric treatment (or other health care) resources available for the parents. A system must be created so that the medical and social services and the other needs of children are provided for and safeguarded while the parent is under treatment and for as long thereafter as needed. It is not at all unlikely that, in addition to the values such a system would have for the children, the very assurance of such concern and care for their children's health and well-being may favorably influence the course of illness of the parents.

In this book the problem is examined, the available resources appraised, and one model of a system which may meet the needs is presented. At the very beginning of the work on which the book is based, the views of the Commissioners of Mental Health, Public Health, and Public Welfare of the Commonwealth of Massachusetts were sought as to the potential significance of the planned research to the responsibilities of their Departments. Each of them welcomed the undertaking and saw potential roles for social workers, public health nurses, and physicians in ambulatory and inpatient medical and psychiatric services in a system of care for children of mentally ill parents. This book will be useful to members of these and other professions and civic leaders who are concerned about children.

William M. Schmidt, M.D.
Professor and Head of Department
of Maternal and Child Health

Introduction

Children of mentally ill parents have received little attention. These studies show that children are exposed to severe and disruptive experiences often resulting in separation and frequent shifts in substitute care; or if they remain at home with a mentally ill parent, they experience a home of turmoil, friction, and inconsistent care and are sometimes physically abused or neglected.

The multiple problems in these families, expecially those related to the children, were infrequently recognized or treated by community health, education, or welfare agencies. Services were fragmented, time-limited, crisis-oriented, and uncoordinated. Suggestions are given regarding methods and organization of services.

Acknowledgements

The studies reported in this volume were carried out with the interest and approval of the following Commissioners of Massachusetts State Departments, to whom the authors extend their thanks:

Dr. Harry C. Solomon, Department of Mental Health
Dr. Alfred L. Frechette, Department of Public Health
Mr. Robert F. Ott, Department of Public Welfare

The authors also wish to express appreciation to the following services and to their representatives and staff, without whom these Studies would not have been possible:

Boston City Hospital, Deputy Commissioners,
Dr. Leon R. Lezer
Leon J. Taubenhaus
Boston City Hospital, Department of Psychiatry,
Dr. Philip Solomon, Director
Dr. Vernon D. Patch
Dr. John B. Sturrock
Boston City Hospital, Sanatorium Division,
Dr. David S. Sherman
Boston Department of Public Welfare,
Mr. William F. Lally (resigned)
Boston School Department,
Mr. William H. Ohrenberger, Superintendent
Community Agencies of Newton and Quincy, especially the Family Service of Newton and the South Shore Mental Health Center

Massachusetts General Hospital, Department of Psychiatry,
  Dr. Morris E. Chafetz
Medfield State Hospital,
  Dr. Theodore F. Lindberg
Metropolitan State Hospital,
  Dr. William F. McLaughlin
Middlesex Sanatorium,
  Dr. Howard M. Payne (deceased)
North Suffolk Mental Health Center,
  Dr. Raquel Cohen
School Superintendents of Chelsea, Revere, and Winthrop
Social Service Exchange,
  Miss Katherine Toll
Taunton State Hospital,
  Dr. W. Everett Glass

Many thanks are also extended to those who served as Directors of
Studies II and III during temporary periods

  Dr. David M. Kaplan
  Dr. Sylvia G. Krakow

and to the Study III pediatrician

  Dr. Arthur J. Salisbury

and to those who served as research interviewers and demonstration
social workers on the Study staff and whose conscientious and tireless
efforts produced the basic data for this report.

Research Interviewers	Demonstration Social Workers
Mrs. Ruth B. Landfield	Mrs. Charlyne D. Costin
Mrs. Katherine B. Perlman	Miss Carmina M. Gordon
Mrs. Phyllis C. Paskauskas	Mrs. Rachel D. Papo
	Mrs. Elinnan R. Reynolds

As always, no volume is possible without able research assistants and secretaries. To them we also extend our thanks, and especially to

Mrs. Gloria M. Tyler

who ably and persistently guided the secretarial staff through the numerous changes in script.

Finally, we acknowledge two persons, without whom the studies would not have been possible:

Dr. Thomas F. Pugh, Director of Medical Statistics and Research, Massachusetts Department of Mental Health

who originally raised the question which was pursued in these studies, and

Dr. William M. Schmidt, Professor and Head of Department of Maternal and Child Health, Harvard School of Public Health

who directed and guided the three studies throughout the 9 years, without whose leadership, support, and interest the studies could not have been completed.

1

The Problem

The twentieth century has been called the "Age of the Child" because of society's concern that its children have opportunity for full physical, emotional, and social development. Early in the century, public concern was focused on problems of child labor which resulted in the enactment of important laws to protect children from hazards affecting their health, education, and general welfare. Group centers for children needing care away from their own homes were developed rather than large congregate institutions. New programs for foster home care for children approximating as nearly as possible the strengths of a family home became later the more usual pattern of substitute care for children. With a clearer understanding of the causation of juvenile delinquency, jails for children awaiting court action were replaced by the establishment of reception centers. Eventually special court sessions for children were organized in many communities. The rise of the juvenile court system provided a method for the study and treatment of the child, rather than the use of punishment. Child psychiatry greatly influenced this and other programs for children and contributed valuable understanding of the child's emotional needs to all professional groups as well as to parents and the public.

Thus, new emphases appeared in our community services for children, and efforts were developed to try to prevent those negative experiences for children that contributed to their inability to live normal and happy lives. Basic needs of children and families for food, shelter, and clothing, and more recently for medical care have at last become recognized by society, but society has not yet made adequate provisions for these needs in families unable to do so themselves. Even though Federal legislation has at last been passed to provide minimum maintenance for children and families in need, there continue to be many families without adequate support. This is worse in some areas than in other areas. More needs to be done for children, but the twentieth century can be recognized as the age when public concern for the welfare of its children was awakened, services and legislation were strengthened, and there was some reduction in the more serious effects of poverty, ill health, inadequate child care, unsafe and inappropriate working conditions, lack of play, and limited schooling. In spite of this, there are still children living in deprivation in this rich country.

Much has been written about the needs of children for adequate care, protection, schooling, and preparation for adult life. With the emphasis on the child's emotional development, attention has been drawn to his need for loving care by a mother or mother substitute and the dangers when consistent care is interrupted for various reasons. Studies have been made of the effects on the child's social and psychological adjustment when he is separated from the mother and family. Studies have also been made of the effect of separation of the child from his family because of the child's own need for hospitalization or other institutional care. Well-known studies by Bowlby, Fries, Anna Freud, Robinson, Spitz, and others have shown that there may be severe emotional deprivation when a child is separated from his mother by being institutionalized. Additional separations for the older child also occur when he is separated from his family including those from siblings, peer groups, and schoolmates. Thus, the total life of the child may be seriously altered by a separation from his family which makes it necessary for him to adjust to a new way of living.

Furthermore, hospitalization of a child frequently occurs suddenly and with little time to prepare him to understand what is happening. The usual fears and anxieties of parents at such a time are readily transmitted to the child who sees the new experience as one with uncertainties and to be dreaded. Films taken of children experiencing hospitalization, especially those by Robinson in England and Mason in the United States, clearly depict the effect, especially on young children, of separation from parents and the frightening routines and procedures of hospital care.

Problems experienced by children when they themselves are separated from home, not because of their own need for hospital care but because of a parent's need for such care, has had little attention until recently. Yet the impact on children may be even greater, especially when the parent is, in addition, mentally ill. When mental illness of a parent necessitates hospitalization, many disturbances and disruptions in normal family activities are to be anticipated. It is assumed that the children in these families have the same types of risks as other children whose fathers or mothers are absent from the home because of death, divorce, separation, or other reasons; however, these children have also the added risk of having a parent who is mentally ill for a shorter or longer period of time prior to his hospital care, and thereby the children are intimately involved in the disturbances peculiar to mental illness.

With the mental illness of one parent and the emotional strain on the other, children may be deprived of their usual care including ordinary health supervision or adequate medical care. They may be deprived of the familiar surroundings of their own homes, playmates, and schoolroom brought about through abrupt, baffling changes in living arrangements of unknown duration. Their familiar and normal family activities may be invaded and disrupted by caretaking persons who are reluctant, ill-suited, or poorly prepared to cope with the extraordinary demands of this crisis period. Situations such as these are known to exist, but little is known of their extent or severity.

There is some literature directed to the concerns and reactions of the whole family when a member is hospitalized for a mental illness. The excellent series by Clausen, Yarrow, et al. (1955) discussed the impact of mental illness on the family, particularly as it relates to the wife when the husband is hospitalized. Except for an early paper by Treudley (1946) which describes some of the disruptions and disturbances in everyday needs in families of mentally ill parents such as for housing, food, sleep, and care of children, there is very little literature directed primarily to the risks for children when their usual care is interrupted.

A study by Pugh in the Massachusetts Department of Mental Health showed that in 1950, approximately 7,500 persons were admitted to state mental hospitals in Massachusetts. About 1,200 of these admissions were patients between the ages of 15 and 54 years who were married, widowed, divorced, or separated who lived in a household containing one or more children. The hospital records, however, gave little, if any, information about these children or the impact on the family of the hospitalization. Figuring on an average of two children per family, a minimal estimate in a given year would indicate that at least 2,400 children in Massachusetts had a parent who was hospitalized during that year because of mental illness. This raises the question of what care these children received, what additional problems were created for them because of the hospitalization of their parents, and whether the substitute care was adequate. The hospitals to which these parents were admitted had no answers to these questions.

Historically, the mental hospital was the resource for the mentally ill. It was essentially a custodial setting for what was then considered an incurable disease involving progressive deterioration. The hospital was designed to separate the patient from his family and the community for an indefinite period. This concept of the mental hospital as the primary resource for the mentally ill is changing, but the lag between the original and newer concept of care is still considerable. However, the responsibility for the care of children of mentally ill parents has not been assumed by the hospitals providing care for the parents but by the community child-welfare agencies when they received requests for placement.

There have been dramatic changes in the pattern of hospitalization of patients with mental illness which have created different problems in the care of children. Child-welfare agencies are recognizing that the placement of the children of the mentally ill in foster homes, for example, is presenting difficulties because of the briefer period of the parent's hospitalization and because of the tendency for patients to be readmitted to hospitals within a relatively short period of time. For example, in one of the hospitals in our study, 75% of all new admissions were discharged after three months hospitalization and many of these patients were readmitted within another three months. This trend toward shorter periods of hospitalization is typical in many mental hospitals throughout the country. Another significant trend is reflected in the admission of a broader segment of the population. Alcoholics, for example, represent 30 to 40% of new admissions. Depressed patients and those with neuroses, personality disorders, or acute situational disturbances constitute a greater proportion of the patients hospitalized than in the past.

Specialization and poor communication patterns between agencies result in the fragmentation of services provided the family. It is still unusual, for example, for a child-welfare agency responsible for the care of a child to be informed, much less consulted, by a state hospital about the admission or discharge plan for the parent.

Hospitalization of the mental patient is now viewed as a relatively brief phase of what, hopefully, will become a continuous, comprehensive care program of the mentally ill, having its primary focus in the community. The hospital in this system of organization would be integrated into a community network of services as one of many resources for the treatment, control, and rehabilitation of a patient and his family. This plan is more a hope than a reality at this time, but there is evidence to suggest that such comprehensive care is a goal that may eventually be achieved.

For these reasons, the studies reported in this volume were carried out by the Department of Maternal and Child Health of the Harvard School of Public Health with the financial assistance of the Charles H.

Hood Dairy Foundation, the Rosenthal Foundation, and the National Institutes of Mental Health. They were designed to investigate a sample of families with a mentally ill parent to determine the kind and severity of child-care problems; to analyze the types of problems already existing in these families or those created by the calamity of mental illness of a parent; to determine the needs that are being met effectively through normal or organized resources; and to pinpoint, if possible, ways of so organizing our community services of health and welfare that children and families may receive the help they need during the crises of care for mental illness and in the long period of reassimilation of the ill parent into the family and the community. Efforts to identify those periods in the course of such crises when help can be most effective and thus prevent some of the impact of the illness and separation on children could contribute toward lessening or preventing some of the hazards to children and their long-time effects on children's chances for healthy development. The studies reported in this volume, therefore, will shed light on these points and will suggest possible ways that services can be developed to help families and children at these periods of crisis in their lives.

2

The History

The twentieth century, in its increasing interest in children, has given special attention to the effect on children of various experiences. Up to now more attention in the literature has been directed to the reactions of children when they are separated from home and family than when they remain in their own homes and are separated from parents because the parents are the ones who leave the home. Some of the early studies, however, which report the reactions of children when they are separated for their own hospitalization or institutional care, are of interest as a background to this study which is primarily concerned with what happens to children of mentally ill parents when the children are separated from ill parents or are exposed to the ill mother at home.

The following references are a sample of the literature on children separated from parents, the family and family functioning, children of mentally ill parents, psychiatric services, emergency services, and homemaker services. Not all the available literature has been encompassed within this limited review. The papers cited have been chosen to present the thinking of other writers in regard to many of the problem areas described in this volume. Many of these references contain bibliographies that supplement the references in this chapter. Many of the well-established writings with which the reader is undoubtedly familiar have not been included.

Children Separated from Mothers

The term "hospitalism" was used by Freund (1910). The clinical picture and high fatality rate were ascribed to two factors: infection and inadequate knowledge of artificial feeding. A pediatrician, Chapin (1915), summarized various reports showing high fatality rates in institutions for infants and this laid the bases for the later development of foster home care. The idea that in addition to infection and improper feeding, other factors were involved soon emerged (Brennemann, 1932). Infection was still considered a major factor, but "hospitalization is not wholly coextensive with parenteral infection." The idea emerged that an absence of mothering was an important element and therefore that babies should be picked up, carried about, amused, and "mothered." Like Brennemann's report, loneliness in infants was described as the basis of close and careful clinical observation by a pediatrician, Bakwin (1942). In this paper, Bakwin gives a good review of the reports cited above and others (including some animal studies) and reports the opening of the wards at the Bellevue Hospital in New York City to more parental visiting and more "mothering care" of infants.

Ribble (1943) speculates extensively in regard to infant behavior. She insisted that infant's respiration could not be established unless they are fondled, held, and given the possibility of "sucking freely." She stated that such failure to establish proper respiration resulted in poor speech development, delay in talking, and possibly even impaired physical and mental health. Ribble gives one case vignette of a highly disturbed broken family. She dedicates her book, however, to all inquiring parents and speculates about the dire risks if an infant is handled too little, or allowed to cry too long.

Bakwin's second paper (1949) on emotional deprivation presents a more detailed clinical picture of the reaction to deprivation among institutionalized infants. In this he makes the important point that children reared at home who show pallor, quietness, and motor retardation, which are associated with emotional deprivation, are likely to be more adversely affected in hospitals because they tend to be left alone, while livelier babies get most of the attention. This report provides a fuller review of earlier papers, and calls attention to the practice in a New Zealand hospital of admitting mothers to hospitals with their babies requiring operations (Pickerill, C., 1947).

Studies by Spitz (1945) and Spitz and Wolf (1946) provide clinical descriptions of infants in the age range 6 to 12 months, separated from their mothers. The infant's "anaclitic depression" is manifested by the withdrawal from the environment to the extent of rejecting the environment, apprehension of others who attempt to approach him, sadness, insomnia, loss of weight, and loss of appetite. In addition, the infant was often found to be inert, stuperous, and sometimes retarded in developmental activity.

Studies by Burlingham and Freud (1942, 1943) explored the problems of a group of English children left homeless during the Second World War. It was found that regressive behavior was most marked in the age group between 1½ and 2½ years, as contrasted with the 3 years and upward age groups.

Bowlby's monograph (1951) contributed information about the dangers of gross maternal deprivation. Clinical observations were projected into a world health outlook (which was mostly, however, limited to Europe) as Bowlby described the connection between conditions in the world and the deprivation of children. He mentioned physical or mental illness of the parent as conditions to be regarded as a potential source of deprivation for children, particularly when the natural home group was intact and not functioning effectively, or when the natural home group needed to be divided. This monograph, subtitled "A Contribution to the U.N. Programme for the Welfare of Homeless Children," is mainly devoted to a review of the effects of institutional life. Bowlby drew two inferences that were subject to later modifications:

1) ". . . when deprived of maternal care, the child's development is almost always retarded physically, intellectually and socially—and that

symptoms of physical and mental illness may appear."

2) ". . . children thrive better in bad homes than in good institutions." The child may be "ill-fed and ill-sheltered, he may be dirty and suffering from disease, he may be ill-treated, but unless his parents have wholly rejected him, he is secure in the knowledge that there is someone to whom he is of value and who will strive, even though inadequately, to provide for him until such time as he can fend for himself." This statement was later modified: "It all depends on how bad is the home and how good the institution."

In Appendix 4 Bowlby gives figures on children deprived of a normal home life (probably admitted to institutions or foster care). He shows in a Swedish series that mental and physical illness of a parent accounts for 23% of the cases placed away from home; in one British series, 25%; and in one U.S. and one British, 6 and 9%, respectively.

Bowlby's generalizations made a great impact throughout the western world at least on the agencies providing services to children and they still have their carry-over as will be shown by examining agencies' services in this Study. They were later, in 1962, amended when the World Health Organization published a series on Maternal Deprivation: A Reassessment by Ainsworth (1962). These papers amended the oversimplifications in the Bowlby monograph and contributed more specific definitions of deprivation to include hidden or qualitative deprivation, classification of factors influencing the degree of damage to children resulting from depriving separation experiences, and the possibility of reversal of such damage. Ainsworth states that a problem theoretically and practically important is the extent to which the "major mother figure can or should share her responsibilities with other figures, with or without continuity, in order to discover those patterns (and there are probably several) which are optimal for the child's development of identification, security, and subsequent mental health." This is more germane to the problems of children of mentally ill parents reported in this volume than is Bowlby's concentration on "the family" as almost the only acceptable form of care.

Whereas Bolwby's concern was with maternal deprivation, Ainsworth pointed out the need to examine the father's relation to the infant and young child and the effects of different types of paternal care. This is especially important in the families with mentally ill parents.

In this series of Public Health Papers, Prugh and Harlow, writing of "Masked Deprivation" say that misplaced emphasis on Bowlby's earlier statements lead to the facile, erroneous conclusion that the child's own home is always better than a foster home or institution. "Masked Deprivation" can have equally devastating effects as more gross maternal deprivation. The child's response to separation is a complex process. It is affected by its nature, duration, age and stage of development of the child, his emotional conflicts, ego capacity, physical health, and other factors including the reactions of those around him. In this same series Buckle and Labovici emphasized the importance of the family disturbance before and after the separation. One study of delinquent boys and a control group by Andry (1960) showed no differences in maternal deprivation but more disturbed father-child relationships among the delinquent boys.

A study by Aubry (1955) of children placed in an institution near Paris is a part of a series of studies bringing out the multiplicity of caretakers and the impersonal character of nursing care. Among the reasons for placement of children in Aubry's study, only 4 of 147 were for mental illness of a parent. This institution was mainly for short-stay children. Aubry thinks that the children of mentally ill parents present especially difficult problems from her observation.

The Family and Family Functioning

The impact of specific problems on families and family functioning in different crisis situations has been described by Koos (1946) and Hill (1949). The incidence and interrelationships of the four major human problems of dependency, ill health, maladjustment, and recreational needs have been studied by Buell and associates (1952) who found, in the community studied, that while community services have been multiplying rapidly, they fail to meet these major needs in a coordinated and purposeful direction.

Study within the psychiatric field indicates growing concern with the family of the psychiatric patient as central to understanding and treatment of the patient himself. Spiegel and Bell (1959) offer a comprehensive statement of the problem of bridging psychoanalytic theory and sociological theory in conceptualizing patient and family interaction in a new "transactional" approach. Albert (1960) illustrates this approach in a theoretical formulation of three stages of disruptive interaction between patient and family which could lead to possible prediction of illness and consequent selective use of mental hospitals and other community and social resources for treating patients and families. Freeman and Simmons (1963) in a broad survey of discharged mental patients stressed family composition as one of a wide range of factors which determine improvement. Hollingshead and Redlich (1958), in their classic study of social class and mental illness, indicate that education and occupation are social determinants both in mental illness itself and in the help-seeking patterns that derive from it.

In order to estimate the significance of certain circumstances in family histories as etiological factors in psychoneurosis, Ingham (1949) at Los Angles studied a group of patients so diagnosed in the neurophychiatric clinic of the Student Health Service at the University of California at Los Angeles and compared this group to a group of control students at the same university. He found twelve factors to which family circumstances were more frequent in the neuroses including mental illness in one or both parents. In the clinical group 47.1% reported at least one mentally ill patient as opposed to 2.7% of the control. The results indicated that mental illness in some member of the family and intrafamily conflict were important concomitants of neurosis. The following conclusions were suggested by the data: mental illness in parents, separation of parents, lack of adjustment between them, rejection of parent figures, parental overrestriction, mental illness in siblings or disturbed relationships between them, and disruption of the subject's marriage, are indicated considerably more frequently in those students suffering from psychoneuroses than in the university population at large.

Agencies

In a clarifying paper Hill (1958) presents a scheme for depicting the interplay of stress or event, contributing hardships, and family resources in producing a family crisis. Surrounding family inadequacy, he includes cultural diversity, conflicting roles, economic and other pressures, class-membership pressures, unrealized aspirations, and inadequate interpersonal relationships. He discusses the implications for services emphasizing that they should be neighborhood oriented.

It is noteworthy that those families that best succeeded in meeting the crisis of wartime separation made frequent mention of the accessibility of relatives, neighbors and friends. They rarely mentioned . . . the churches, the family agencies, or other welfare groups. . . . As we have seen the need . . . help might often have consisted simply of providing an opportunity to ventilate their anxieties, share their woes and ask for reassuring, simple advice about problems occasioned by the absence of the husband or father, or the changed regulations for children attending schools in double shifts. There are, at the present time, few agencies to which families willingly turn for help on the more superficial levels of life.

He further urges that professional services be given with the total family context in mind, serving the child's family as a family rather than serving the child solely as a personality. He concludes that counseling and case work become "patchword remedies" unless a strong program of preventive social work and education is undertaken by agencies. He believes that to exercise family leadership will require different preparation of social workers.

Children of Mentally Ill Parents

An article by Truedley (1946) describing some disruptions and disturbances in every day needs of housing, food, sleep, and care of children of mentally ill parents, seems particularly pertinent. Her statement, "A great deal of thought has been devoted to the mentally ill member in a family but relatively little consideration has been given to the rest of the family who must live with him" is esentially as true today as it was in 1946 when the article was written. Truedley's article suggests the way in which the illness of a parent might effect his ability to fit into normal household routines because of symptoms of withdrawal, aggressiveness, or a tendency to project discomfort upon his home and surroundings.

The series of articles by Clausen and Yarrow (1955) emphasized particularly the impact of mental illness on the marital role and outlined the families' process of defining and dealing with the illness, as well as the relationship of family members to each other, the patient, the hospital, and society.

In addition to continuing studies of childhood development and maternal deprivation of the kind cited earlier, there has been recent literature on the specific area of the current study—children of the mentally ill. Radinsky (1961), a social worker, surveys the changing field of child placement when a parent is mentally ill. New forms of treatment resulting in earlier discharge can adversely affect the child's return home unless the mental health of the family as a unit, as well as the needs of the child, are both skillfully evaluated and treated. She says, "We must come to terms with our recognition of the significance to the child of his own family, for which there is no true substitute and our awareness that there are some families that without help cannot provide a healthy environment for their child."

Sobel's study (1961) of the children of two schizophrenic parents indicated that the babies reared by such parents developed clear-cut signs of depression and irritability in infancy that seem to be at least partially related to parental behavior. The children raised in foster homes seemed to be faring somewhat better.

McClellan (1962) in a comparison study of school records showed that

... children whose mothers had an initial admission to mental hospitals in Massachusetts during the child's first year of life were not shown to be significantly different, at about 12 years of age, from other children. There were hints, however, that their school performance, particularly that of children whose mothers were diagnosed as schizophrenic, was somewhat inferior.

The study presented has relevance to current interest in certain problems which arise when the mother of an infant requires hospitalization for mental illness. Should the infant be brought into hospital with its mother? If separation of child from mother in such circumstances is to occur by choice or necessity, what efforts should be made, if any, to offer even tentative answers to these questions on the basis of this exploratory study? It would be hazardous to infer from our findings that exposure of very young children to maternal mental illness carries little risk of psychological damage to the children. On the other hand, it is conceivable that genetic rather than environmental or chance factors might have caused the differences noted between the study and comparison groups.

Doniger (1962) describes an English study in which the mentally ill, hospitalized patient and spouse were questioned on various aspects of family life and relationships within the family, with special reference to children. It was concluded that many of the children might require psychiatric help in their own right and that such help could well be given at the point of the mother's hospitalization. This paper emphasizes that grossly disturbed mothers can be more harmful than suitable substitutes in caring for their children. Doniger also emphasizes that psychiatric hospital care is naturally patient-centered, but that mothers should be treated from a family standpoint. She discusses community organization to achieve the experience gained in admitting children with their mothers to a psychiatric hospital. She sees this as reinforcing a concept of family, rather than patient-oriented care.

Sussex (1963) and Sussex, Gassman, and Raffel (1963) discuss a preliminary study of latency aged children whose psychotic mothers are being treated while in the home. It was found that family resources supported or substituted for the mothering role when this primary role was disrupted by illness. It was found that impairment in the mothering role due to mental illness and absence of such supplementary family resources does, indeed, affect children unfavorably. The article stresses the need to evaluate carefully those factors that may influence the emotional impact on children of the presence of an acutely psychotic mother when she is at home during treatment. These factors include the mother's preservation of mothering capacity, the degree to which the father or other available adult can support the mother in continuing her role, the capacity of the father or another available adult to substitute mothering if the mother can no longer do so, the child's own resources for coping successfully with the emotional crisis, the economic situation of the family, and the attitudes of the subculture in which the family lives. It was found that as long as the mothering capacity exists, the mother's continued presence in the home is positive to the children and neglect of physical services to them leads to no harm. It was suggested that in schizophrenic mothers, their distortions may confuse the children and lead to hospitalization as a preferred method of treatment. It was suggested that a decision as to whether to treat the mother in the home or to hospitalize her should include evaluation of the father and other significant adults, of the children, and of the social setting in which the family lives.

Cowie (1961) studied the incidence of neurosis in 330 children of mentally ill parents and compared these controls. The mean ages were 19.6 and 19.8 years, respectively. There was slightly more neuroticism among the children of mentally ill patients than of controls. More children of mentally ill parents developed their neurotic behavior within two years of onset of parental illness than was expected.

Boardman (1963) in discussing the problem of neglected and battered children states that criteria are desperately needed to differentiate the parents who can be helped to act responsibly from those who cannot. Services must be provided to those parents who can utilize them and effective means must be employed to insure that the child's health is not grossly damaged if the parents cannot utilize the services. This is in sharp contrast to Bowlby's statement in the monograph which indicated that a child may be sick, dirty, or abused but if he has his own mother he is well supported.

Buckle (1965) further states that parental deprivation is pathogenic, leading to many typical disturbances in children. There is evidence to support the idea that a child's disturbance following neglect by his mother is due to the family disturbance that precedes and follows the neglect rather than to the deprivation itself.

Psychiatric Services

New trends and patterns in relation to the problem of mental illness were both reflected in and initiated by the work of the first Joint Commission on Mental Illness and Health in the United States. The excellent reports of this first study in the history of the mental health of the country states (1961):

The objective of modern treatment of persons with major mental illness is to enable the patient to maintain himself in the community in a normal manner. To do so, it is necessary (1) to save the patient from the debilitating effects of institutionalization as much as possible, (2) if the patient requires hospitalization, to return him to home and community life as soon as possible, and (3) thereafter to maintain him in the community as long as possible. Therefore, after-care and rehabilitation are essential parts of all service to mental patients, and the various methods of achieving rehabilitation should be integrated in all forms of services, among them day hospitals, night hospitals, after-care clinics, public health nursing services, foster family care, convalescent nursing homes, rehabilitation centers, work services, and ex-patient groups.

Recent literature, especially Bellak (1960) and Detre (1963), demonstrates these trends in a new role for the general hospital, home care of psychiatric patients by Friedman (1960), and cooperative patterns between mental hospitals and community agencies by Smith (1960) and Coleman (1967). British and Canadian experience, stimulated by new patterns of governmental responsibility, follow similar trends [Freeman (1963) and McNair (1961)].

In Crocetti's paper (1963), which reported a study of opinions of a population in Baltimore with respect to home care for the mentally ill, the authors point out that it is not just a matter of determining whether people are willing to care for the mentally ill at home, but of determining (1) whether such care is advantageous to the mentally ill, and (2) whether the mental patient can remain at home without disturbing interpersonal relations and thus avoid harming the structure of the family and/or neighborhood groups.

Freeman and Simmons (1961) studied treatment experiences of patients after discharge from a mental hospital. Treatment and help-seeking experiences of patients and their families failed to show that recent changes advocated in hospital regime and release practices had been accompanied by programs which effectively extended the therapeutic process into the community or included families of patients as parts of a broadened treatment base.

In Friedman's study (1960) of sixty patients provided home treatment instead of hospitalization, 60% remained in the community after the first 15 months of the study. However, he reported that several children in these families were found to be very disturbed. Obtaining treatment for them had been difficult in the past because of the parents' inability to cooperate. In these families, because of episodic crises and the need to prevent hospitalization, home care with visits of doctor, nurse, or social worker sustained the family.

Hoenig (1965) gives the results of a four-year follow-up study of a stratified sample of new patients at a general hospital psychiatric clinic in Manchester, England. His study covers diagnoses, referral, disposition, length of stay, mortality, morbidity, vocational and social rehabilitation, burden on the patient's family and household, and attitudes of patients and relatives toward the extramural service.

Lemkau and Crocetti (1961) described the postcare program organized by Dr. Arie Querido, founder of the Amsterdam Municipal Psychiatric Service. The program includes medical supervision through home and office visits, adequate housing, and work. The goal is realistic management in terms of life in the community. In the area of work, the aim is to keep the patient employed as frequently and as long as possible rather than permanent placement.

Deane (1963) at the Vermont State Hospital also emphasizes the constructive use of employment to handle psychotic tendencies. Other methods used include continuity of relationship between patients and hospital personnel, such as home and work visits, contact with other former patients, the role of the rehabilitation house, and short-term return to the hospital on a temporary or day-or-night basis.

Emergency Services

The traditional utilization of hospital emergency services mainly for medical crises has been changing rapidly in the past few years. It is stated in a study by Bergman and Haggerty (1962), "In most hospitals today the traditional concept of the emergency room as a receiving ward for the accidentally injured and critically ill patients, no longer holds." A paper by Weinerman and Edwards (1954) states,

The role of the general hospital has changed from that of a last resort for the seriously ill to a community resource for a broad spectrum of general medical care services to ambulatory patients. As medical practice has become more specialized, more highly structured and less personal, physicians are not as readily available for sudden calls and not as willing to handle a wide variety of acute problems.

In Coleman's report (1963) of "The General Hospital Emergency Room and Its Psychiatric Problems," he discusses eight suggestions as to what kinds of patients with psychiatric problems come to the emergency services, why they come at the particular time, and what they hope to achieve by their visit. One of his suggestions states that,

In some instances, probably a good many, crises arise when the patient has been experiencing over a period of time certain kinds of manipulative, extruding rejections by other family members, or is unable to reach persons on whom he might otherwise depend during crisis periods. The phenomenon of "alienation," as a sociological concept, runs parallel to that of "depression," "depersonalization," or "derealization," as psychiatric states. Often, such reactions seem to be associated with changes in the structure of the family, as for example when a key person has died, or when other crucial experiences such as marriage, pregnancy, childbirth, or illness disrupt the dynamic stability of a family group, or at least of the group on which the patient has been accustomed to rely for his sense of social support. These are people who are more than ordinarily vulnerable to stress.

In a national survey of hospital emergency services, Skudder and his associates (1961) reported an increase in the proportions of "non-urgent" cases by patients with "ordinary" medical care needs. He estimated that 42% of the patients in emergency services were nonurgent cases while accidental injuries comprised about one-third of the total.

Although the proportions of patients who come to emergency services with real "emergency" or "crisis" conditions have become significantly lessened in recent years because of the use of the emergency services for nonurgent needs, definitions of what constitutes a medical emergency or crisis still remain fairly well established. A definition of a psychiatric emergency has been given by Miller (1959) as "any individual who develops a sudden or rapid disorganization in his capacity to control his behavior or to carry out his usual personal, vocational and social activities. A psychiatric emergency thus refers to the behavior of an individual rather than to any particular category of psychiatric illness."

The psychiatric "emergency" or "crisis," and the type and extent of community resources available, or not available, to handle it is becoming an ever increasing concern, particularly of physicians, psychiatrists, and social workers. New approaches to meet these concerns have been introduced in a variety of settings. One approach has been that of the Psychiatric Home Treatment Service developed by Friedman (1960) et al. The Service is based in a state mental hospital, utilizing a psychiatric team of psychiatrist and social worker who make home visits in response to a report of a psychiatric crisis or serious mental disturbance. This approach was introduced as a "neighborhood" based facility since only those families who lived within specifically defined geographic areas adjacent to the state hospital were accepted. Their approach "was to provide better management of mental illness at a time of stress and to see if appropriate alternatives to hospitalization might be possible." Of the sixty patients referred in the first 15 months of operation, 60% were able to remain in the community through prompt evaluation of the patients in their own homes, thereby avoiding unnecessary hospitalizations.

A new approach developed within a municipal general hospital in New York City in 1958 was that of Bellak's (1960) "Trouble Shooting Clinic" which was "designed to offer first-aid to emotional problems. However, unlike the ordinary emergency room, it is not limited only to urgent crises . . . anyone may walk in and simply talk things over," and appointments are not needed. Although most cases were handled in one interview within the clinic itself, occasionally two or three additional visits were made. This was possible because "the staff has acquired certain special techniques in brief psychotherapy. In this way they could handle what could not be done in the overburdened and overcrowded emergency rooms of general hospitals." Bellak states that,

More and more it is becoming recognized that psychiatry has a role to play not only as a basic medical science and as a field of therapeutics, but also as a proper branch of public health and preventive medicine. In this frame of reference, it is only natural that the general hospital should add to the various roles in which it serves the community: that of becoming a nodal point of preventive medicine and public health functions in psychiatry.

Another approach was that of Strickler (1965) et al. who established a community-based Walk-In Center developed from their concern that

much present-day psychotherapy as offered in highly structured conventional treatment facilities makes it difficult for many patients who need help to receive it. The person who is found eligible and receives treatment is usually the highly motivated person, in the upper or middle income group, relatively well educated, and psychologically sophisticated. Many individuals in the community, however, do not desire or require the kind of traditional treatment offered. For them, there are few community resources.

The Benjamin Rush Center for Problems of Living in Los Angeles is described as a psychiatric clinic that does not have the usual trappings of one and is based on the general approach of Bellak's "Trouble Shooting Clinic." It was "carefully designed to appeal to as diversified a group as possible, including people who in our view are in need of psychiatric care but not likely to seek it." They go on to state, "Emergency psychiatric facilities, offering immediate and brief services do exist, usually in hospitals, but they limit intake to clinical emergencies such as suicide, homicide, and acute psychotic decompensation." This is in opposition to the emergency services utilized in our study, for patients seen in the emergency services of the two general hospitals, because they needed or felt they needed emergency care, were not limited to those with such clinical emergencies as suicide, homicide, or acute psychotic decompensation.

Another statement from Skudder's Survey (1961) of Hospital Emergency Facilities and Services indicates,

What was once the "accident room" designed to handle acute emergency problems in trauma, is now regarded, at least by the general public, as the appropriate initial source of medical care for a wide variety of medical, surgical, pediatric, and even psychiatric problems. The resulting increase in emergency room visits has been shown to exceed 400 percent in many hospitals and, in some, to exceed prewar levels by 600 percent. It is obvious that this increased use of emergency facilities by the general public indicates a basic shift in patterns of medical care.

Coleman (1963), in discussing the reasons why patients present themselves to emergency services, states,

Many emotionally disturbed persons need, or believe they need, immediate medical attention. There seems little doubt that psychiatric problems are contributing their share to the increased use of hospital emergency, the criteria often being based upon the severity of symptoms or of behavioral deviations. . . . It has been suggested that more time is spent with "pseudo" psychiatric emergencies than with clear-cut problems.

In addition, therefore, to large increases in emergency service visits, it seems obvious that more and more patients are presenting problems within social and family-life stress situations which may or may not be crises or emergencies. The presenting problems include those stress components within their marital situations, difficulties in child-rearing and parent-child relationships, conflicts derived from unwanted pregnancies or childbirth, economic difficulties, and many others, whether they are superimposed upon an existing psychiatric component or not.

Weinerman and associates at Yale (1966) in a study of determinants of use of hospital emergency services state that the emergency service is a basic source of medical care for the economically depressed inner-city population and the back-up resource for the self-supporting community when private care is unavailable. The population using the emergency facility at Yale is young, male, unmarried, central urban, and relatively poor. At times of perceived crisis, the majority of persons of all classes who use the emergency service tend to go there directly without medical referral. The most pressing need is for a community system of medical care which will make personal, continuous, and comprehensive health service available to all classes in the population.

Ungerleider (1960) at University Hospitals in Cleveland studied the Psychiatric Emergency Consultation Service for a period of 6 months in 1958 during which time 378 psychiatric emergencies were seen. Most of these were as outpatients. Over half of the patients were female, white, Protestant, and married. The maximum frequency was in the 30-39 year old range. Half of the patients had not been to the University Hospitals before. Positive and specific history of past psychiatric illness was given by 23% of the patients; about 17% had been or were currently being treated in the outpatient department at University Hospitals. The duration of the presenting problem extended from an acute problem arising on the same day for 36% to over a year for 7%. In 82% of the cases no medications were administered. Follow-up showed that 15% did not follow recommendations; 11% were unavailable. In 52% hospitalization was recommended but in only 43% did the patients become hospitalized.

At the Bronx Municipal Hospital, Coleman (1959) established an emergency psychiatric clinic which sees patients on a 24 hour basis and which offers immediate treatment as well as referral. Brief therapy is instituted immediately in many acute neurotic and psychotic decompensations. Coleman believes that there are many more cases of acute neurotic and psychotic decompensation in the community than had previously been thought. Immediate consultations are also provided social agencies in emergencies and thus they are more able to cope with a broader range of community mental health problems.

Homemaker Service

Stewart, Pennell, and Smith (1958) of the Public Health Service and

Social Security Administration published a directory of homemaker services and a pamphlet describing Homemaker Services (1958) which included all agencies in the United States with a homemaker. Homemaker services were orignially started in relation to the needs of families when mothers were hospitalized for a physical condition, especially childbirth, in order to keep the children at home and the family intact. In more recent years interest has swung to the use of homemaker services for mentally and chronically ill and aged. The general purposes of homemaker services are:

1) As a preventive to ill-considered or unsatisfactory placement of children
2) As a support in efforts to maintain the family enabling the parent to work out a home care plan for children
3) As an aid to the patient's own psychiatric rehabilitation.

Homemaker services have been developed under a variety of auspices and within various kinds of agencies. The particular emphasis of a homemaker services is determined by the auspices under which the service is given. Thus, homemaker service in the Children's Aid Society, New York City, utilize homemakers for diagnostic purposes in assessing children's problems; for meeting children's needs when parents neglect their function through incompetence or illness; for protective service to children; and for relieving the burdened parent. In this setup the homemaker service is seen as a separate service within the agency but very closely related to the counseling and foster care programs of the agency. When homemaker service is set up under a Visiting Nurse Agency, the homemaker is utilized in relation to medical planning and is used to help the patient assume responsibility for following medical recommendations.

The Public Assistance homemaker services are more connected with the needs of a financially dependent group. The Cook County program has utilized homemakers' time in a very flexible way in some AFDC cases. The New York City Department of Welfare homemaker service has a particularly interesting aspect of supervision, in that field workers are used as supervisors of the homemakers—each field person being responsible for a group of eight or nine homemakers; "on the job" supervision affords direct and responsible contact with the actual home situations and provides a more central kind of liaison with the total agency.

The literature is replete with illustrations of the length of time and the extent of study necessary in order to initiate, strengthen, and interpret homemaker services regardless of auspices.

The New Jersey experience illustrates how a State Health Department can stimulate local communities to develop homemaker service and can take leadership in setting up training for the homemakers at the State University. In considering the administration of homemaker services, attention is given to:

1) Employment practices, including the selection of homemakers. It is thought that there is a large group of women available for this kind of job if recruiting is properly done.

2) Relationships between homemaker and other staff members (particularly in family agencies).

3) Training given at Rutgers includes such content as family and community relationships, safety and accident prevention, food and nutrition, understanding of children and the elderly, patient relationships, understanding of mental illness, and occupational therpy. It is expected that the persons recruited would have some familiarity with and skills in the general service which they are asked to perform. This includes personal care, cleaning, laundry, preparation and meal-serving, leisure-time activities, sewing, mending, and helping the children with homework. Thus the training is geared to the understanding of the purposes of homemaker service for family and community, and geared also to the maintenance of standards of home care and child rearing.

Pennell and Smith (1959) in their analysis of families served by homemakers in the National Study showed that seven of ten families required assignment of a homemaker because the children's mother was in a medical institution or was dead. In several instances, a sick mother at home was unable to care for her children. Slightly more than half the families in the study received homemaker service through voluntary family or family and child care agencies, about 30% through departments of public welfare and the balance from independent, voluntary homemaker agencies, visiting nurse associations, or health agencies. Half of the families had service for at least 3 months; 4% of the families had been served by a homemaker for 5 years or longer. Homemakers were often assigned to care for children for 8 hours a day, 5 days a week. One-third of the families with children had about 40 hours of homemaker's time during the study week. Half of the families had less care than this. Resident or live-in service is infrequent, since relatives, neighbors, and friends can usually be counted on to supplement the homemaker's hours. Mental, psychoneurotic, and personality disorders were listed as the fifth reason for using homemakers.

Among those families with ill or diaabled persons at home, the major reason for the assignment of a homemaker was to provide long-term care to enable the patient to remain out of the hospital, nursing home, or other type of institution. About six out of ten families had long-term homemaker assignments. Short-term homemaker assignments were provided to one third of the families, and was more usual among families with children. The number of homemakers currently employed is small, and expansion of homemaker services is needed.

Margolis (1957) traces the development of visiting homemaker services with special note of the Chicago Home for the Friendless. He uses case histories to illustrate the following functions of homemakers: substitute for ill or deceased mother; as part of a therapeutic team helping a mentally ill mother before, during, and after hospitalization;

aiding overwhelmed mothers; giving personal and psychological support to the elderly in maintaining their homes; and as observer to help the team diagnose and evaluate the home situation.

The Ross Laboratories (1965) reports a demonstration project at the Evansville, Indiana State Hospital of the value of homemaker services provided by a mental hospital to patients and their families. Five homemakers trained by the hospital personnel in the hospital setting are full-time employees of the Social Service Department. The project was undertaken because the hospital staff became aware of the difficulty of treating a mother who was worried about her children during her hospitalization and of the feelings of loss and trauma engendered in the children by the mother's absence. The homemakers are trained by the hospital and are carefully supervised. Their time in any one home is limited to a maximum of 6 months.

The paper also discusses protection of children by providing foster care for those who have psychotic mothers at home, the related problems of child abuse, and ends with: "A family in the crisis of mental illness often needs several kinds of services. If these are to by provided a system of interagency and interdisciplinary communication must be instituted."

3

The Overview of the Studies

The Department of Maternal and Child Health of the Harvard School of Public Health has been interested in studying risks to mothers and children when there are hazards within their physical or psychosocial environment. The three studies, reported in this volume, have examined the risks to children when one parent was mentally ill.

Questions which prompted the studies were:

1) Are there risks to children in relation to the adequacy of their care when a parent is mentally ill, and is the risk greater when the father or the mother is the ill person?

2) What kinds of risks does the child experience and how severe are they?

3) What are the more usual patterns of substitute care of children and did these differ according to the age of children, which parent was ill, the family income, or the geographical location of the family?

4) To what extent and for what purposes did the families utilize community resources of health and welfare, and how effective were these services when used?

5) How can families who have children at home with a mentally ill parent be identified early in order that these families may have assistance, if needed, with child-care arrangements?

6) What new or different methods of providing services are required to prevent risks to children throughout a parent's illness and its reacerbations?

7) What system of organization or reorganization of resources would meet the needs of these families?

The Three Studies

To seek answers to these questions a series of three studies was carried out. Study I, the Pilot Study, secured the sample of families to be studied from those parents who had been admitted during a certain period of time to one state mental hospital in Massachusetts who had children up to 21 years of age living at home. This hospital drew patients from two small cities and several towns surrounding the hospital. A small number of patients from a second state hospital serving more urban areas was added to the study sample to see what differences there might be between urban and nonurban families in relation to child-care. In order to determine whether there were any differences in the living arrangement and care of children or in the use of community health and social agencies whether the parent was hospitalized for a physical or mental illness, the pilot study included a comparable but smaller group of parents hospitalized in two state tuberculosis sanatoria serving urban and suburban families.

Since Study I showed that there were problems for children when a parent was hospitalized for either a physical or mental illness and that in general families made little use of health and social agencies, a demonstration study, Study II, was carried out. This study was located in another state mental hospital which admitted patients from two small cities and thirteen neighboring towns. Parents admitted during a certain period of time to the hospital with children living at home under 18 years of age and who did not have a primary diagnosis of alcoholism constituted the study group. Patients from the two cities admitted to the hospital were the demonstration families and those from the towns were the controls. The demonstration families were provided services by the community health and social agencies on referral from the Study.

The third study, Study III, was also a demonstration study. Several factors led to the decision to undertake this third study. The families in Studies I and II were residents of towns or small cities, many of whom functioned quite adequately until a crisis interfered when they often turned to relatives, friends, and other informal resources. The pattern of social breakdown, seen so often in urban families, especially in deprived areas, was not conspicuous in the second study. The third study was located in a large urban area with several sections of marked deprivation. The aim of the third study was to help families, if possible, before the mother's mental illness became so severe as to require hospitalization and thus, through case finding at an earlier point than hospital admission, to attempt to prevent the several risks to children when the ill parent was still in the home. Since the illness of mothers had been found in the previous studies to create more serious problems for children, this study was limited to mothers.

For these reasons, mothers with children at home under 18 years of age were identified when they came during a certain period of time to the emergency services of two large urban general hospitals and were seen by the psychiatric services. Patients were randomly assigned to demonstration and control groups. In order to insure continuity of service to the maximum extent possible throughout the study year, demonstration social workers on the Study staff worked intensively with the demonstration families.

Ages of Parents and Children

All three studies included ill parents between 16 and 54 years of age who had children living at home. In Study I children up to 21 years of age living at home were included while in the other two studies only children up to 18 years were included. The older children were not a part of Studies II and III because they had been found in Study I to have different and less critical needs in relation to their care than the younger children.

Data Collection

Data necessary to identify patients for the three studies and to furnish information concerning factors associated with the hospitalization or visit to the emergency psychiatric services were initially obtained from hospital admission books, medical records, and, in the case of Study II, a special form filled out by the admitting nurse for this study. The basic social data concerning the family and children were obtained in a series of home interviews with the family or patient which took place at the time of the study intake and during the subsequent year. In Study I case finding took place 6 weeks following the admission of the patient, and a second and final interview was carried out 6 months after the initial one. In Studies II and III, however, the design called for case finding to be instituted at the point of admission or emergency visit, and for the initial home interview to be completed as soon as possible afterwards. Frequently, delays arose in Study III due mainly to difficulties in locating the patients or finding them at home. Second and third interviews in these two studies were carried out at approximately 4-month and 1-year periods following the initial interview.

The initial interview was usually held with members of the patient's family, or the relative caring for the children in Studies I and II, and always with the patients themselves, most of whom were not hospitalized at the time, in Study III. All interviews were of a semistructured type and were carried out by qualified and experienced social caseworkers. Second and third interviews were conducted in accordance with the same schedule of questions as in the initial interview except for data relating to changes occurring in the intervals.

In Studies II and III supplementary data were obtained from school teachers of study children. Teachers in Study II were requested to fill out a brief schedule designed to obtain information concerning repeated grades, academic progress, and behavioral or other difficulties. In Study III brief interviews, for which a similar schedule was utilized, were held with the teachers.

Other sources of data were the community social and health agencies to which families in the studies were currently known or had been known in the past. A list of these agencies was compiled for each family from information obtained from the Social Service Index as well as from the research interview with the family or patient. In Study III agencies were asked to complete a schedule at the beginning and end of the study year, designed to provide additional information concerning family and children's problems, services provided by the agency, and any difficulty in the family's acceptance of service.

Information concerning the health status of children was obtained as part of the research interview in Studies I and II. However, Study III provided for a physical examination of all study children at home by a pediatrician immediately following the initial research interview and a second examination after the final research interview. Although the initial pediatric examinations were made several months late because of difficulty in obtaining the services of a pediatrician, and some families refused this procedure, examinations were completed on most of the study children. The pediatric data included a list of recommendations and suggested treatment facilities in relation to specific child health problems, which were given to the mother in the form of a letter. The pediatric findings therefore permitted an evaluation not only of the health status of the child, but also of the action taken during the year by the family in following up on the initial recommendations.

The Demonstrations

The demonstrations in Studies II and III were designed to provide a planned program of services to mitigate or prevent social and health problems in one group of study children. In Study II this group included patients living in two small cities served by the cooperating state hospital. In these cities the social and health agencies, with the assistance of the study staff, organized a community structure for the provision and coordination of immediate and continuous services for 1 year to the families and children in the study. Community committees were established in the two cities, consisting of representatives of those social and health agencies whose services were most likely to be needed. The primary task of these committees was to coordinate over-all community activity and to serve as a policy-making body for the demonstration. To expedite the work of the committees, one agency in each city was chosen as a "pivot" agency. A family agency and a mental health center served as the "pivot" agencies. These agencies, in turn, selected a member of their staffs to serve as coordinator for the demonstration. The coordinator was responsible for assigning demonstration families to an appropriate agency in the community, consulting with agencies concerning the services given to families, and providing continuity and leadership to the work of the community committees. A member of the study staff served as an ex officio member of the committee.

In Study III, on the other hand, the demonstration staff consisted of three full-time, qualified and experienced social workers who were part of the study staff. Each worker was, however, originally expected to operate out of an agency in the study area. These agencies included a community mental health center, a district office of the city welfare department, and the psychiatric outpatient clinic of one of the general hospitals from which some of the study cases were drawn. These assignments were made in order to give the worker an identification with a service agency; to determine which type of agency provided the most effective base for operating such a service; to demonstrate a potential and appropriate expansion of already existing programs; and to compare the type, extent, and effectiveness of different community services. In practice, however, it was soon found that case assignments could not be restricted to families who might normally be served by these agencies or who lived within areas served by them. Identification of the worker with the local agency, therefore, became confusing to the families. Thereafter the workers were shifted to the Harvard School of Public Health, and families saw more clearly that the study and services emanated from that source.

The task of the demonstration workers was to provide an ongoing social casework service for each demonstration family for a 1-year period, with particular emphasis on the social and health needs of children. They were expected to take the initiative in reaching out to the family and in maintaining as regular and continuous a contact as the needs of the family required. At the same time they were expected to coordinate their services with other community resources including the hospitals or clinics where the parents had treatment. In those instances in which special services were required which would not otherwise have been available, such as homemakers, day care, and summer camp, funds from the study were made available. The inclusion of the demonstration workers as part of the staff in Study III, in contrast to Study II, also made it possible to carry out an evaluation of the demonstration effort in accordance with procedures described below.

The Controls

In Study I the families with parents in the sanatoria served as the control families and comparisons were made between these families and those parents in the mental hospital. In Study II all patients were in one state mental hospital; the families of patients who lived in the thirteen towns served by the hospital were the control families while the families of patients who lived in the two small cities were the demonstration families. The control families were not assigned to any agency and received only such services as were ordinarily available to them on their own request. They were interviewed by the Study staff at three points of assessment only for research purposes. In Study III the patients were randomly assigned to demonstration and control groups. As in Study II, both groups were subject to case finding, assessment, and evaluative processes, but only the demonstration families received the social work services of the demonstration workers. All families were interviewed three times during the study year by the research interviewers.

Analysis of the Data

A primary aim of the analysis in all three studies was to present demographic, social, and health data for these families, bearing upon child-care risks. Since hospitalization of a parent was a prerequisite for inclusion of the family in Studies I and II, an initial focus of these studies was on the living arrangements and care of children when a parent was hospitalized. Noted were the separations which the children experienced from the home of the parent. Separations from home for each child were counted, and these were related to child-care experiences and other risk factors. In Study II three crucial indices of the family resources for child-care were emphasized. These included: (1) The persons available to care for the child, i.e., own parent, relatives, friends, neighbors, or employed help; (2) the housing or physical facilities available for child-care; and (3) financial resources. The first index, that of the caretaker role, was further considered in relation to four components: time available to be a caretaker, health factors, adequacy in the child-care role, and willingness to assume and maintain it. Negatives in any of these factors or components, as noted in the research data and in the reports of community agencies, were checked against each other in order to compare the agencies' awareness of problems in these areas with study observations.

Separations of children from their families for various reasons were also noted and counted in Study III. The same was true for the three components considered as the primary indices of family resources for child-care in Study II. The types of problem areas considered relevant to the care, health, and welfare of children, however, were expanded into a group of twenty. As in Study II, negatives in relation to any of these areas, as noted in the agency reports, were checked against those noted in the research data.

The same group of twenty problem areas was used as a basis for the evaluation of the demonstration in Study III. Each demonstration family was rated independently by three qualified and experienced social caseworkers in order to determine: (1) the child-care, health, and social needs of the family and children of the demonstration families as judged by difficulties noted in the several problem areas during the study year; (2) the extent of the demonstration involvement in each of the problem areas during the year; (3) the degree of movement in each area; and (4) the effectiveness of community resources serving the families during the year as reported by the demonstration staff. For the purpose of this evaluation the initial pediatric, agency, and school reports were made available to the raters, along with the social worker's case record. Each team of raters included the person who had been the demonstration worker on the case as one member, while the other two members consisted, in most instances, of two experienced social caseworkers from outside the regular study staff.

Each child who underwent the pediatric examinations in Study III was given a rating by the pediatrician on his or her *over all health status*. In addition, the pediatrician gave each family a *health performance* rating at the end of the year, as an index of the adequacy or completeness of the family's response to his recommendations, based on the health needs of the child at the time of the first examination. Each of these ratings was made on a three-point scale.

The Study Sample

In the three studies there were included 253 families—199 ill mothers and 54 ill fathers—who had a total of 652 children living in the home. In Study I which was started in 1958 and completed in 1960 there were 84 hospitalized parents; 56 were mentally ill and 28 were tuberculous. The children up to 21 years of age numbered 194.

Study II, started in 1961 and completed in 1965, included 99 families with mentally ill parents who were hospitalized with a total of 243 children under 18 years of age.

Study III was done from 1965 through 1967. It included 70 mentally ill mothers who were seen in two psychiatric emergency services. They had 215 children under 18 years of age.

Comparison of the Findings in the Three Studies

Little data is available on the impact of mental illness of a parent on the care of children and families. The findings of these three studies will clarify the extent and severity of the problems and will indicate what communities may need to do to provide the health and social services which are necessary in order to lessen the impact on children of the mental illness of a parent. Studies I, II, and III have been analyzed together to show similarities and differences in problems, child-care needs, family situations, health and social services, and interagency coordination and planning. Contrasts appear between the data in the three studies, especially between the urban and suburban area studies, between the hospitalized and the nonhospitalized patients, between one- and two-parent families, and between father-patients and mother-patients. The consistency in the three studies in relation to the organization, availability, and utilization of community services raises many questions in relation to the readiness and ability of the present organization of health and social services to meet the needs of children in families in crises because of the mental illness of parents.

4

The Families and the Ill Parents

There were 253 families in the three studies (Table 1). Approximately one-third of the families had only the mother in the home while two-thirds had both parents. More mothers (199) were ill than fathers (54). In the two-parent families the fathers were the patients in slightly less than half of the families.

Compared with the statistics of the metropolitan area the proportion of one-parent families in these studies was three times as great in the small cities and towns in Studies I and II and four times as great in the urban population of Study III. There were no black families in Studies I and II. The proportion of black families in the urban study was twice as great as in the metropolitan area.

Two-thirds of the parents were between the ages of 25 and 44 years. One-third was below 25 years and an equal number over 45 years. One-sixth were fathers. They were older than the mothers by 4.9 years. Mothers who had no husbands at home were younger than the ill mothers with husbands in the home. Also the mothers who were hospitalized were older than the mothers who went to the emergency services.

Separation of Parents

Of the 54 mentally ill fathers in Studies I and II, all but five were living with their families at the time they were admitted to the mental hospital. All of the 74 one-parent mentally ill mothers were not living

TABLE 1
Distribution of 253 ill parents in three studies by ill parent,
number of parents in family, race, and type of case

Study, ill parent, and race	Total families				Two			One		
	Both	Per-cent	Demon-stration	Control	Both	Demon-stration	Control	Both	Demon-stration	Control
Study I										
Mothers	54	64	38	16	34	24	10	20	14	6
Fathers	30	36	18	12	30	18	12	-	-	-
Subtotal	84	100	56	28	64	42	22	20	14	6
Study II										
Mothers	75	76	30	45	53	15	38	22	15	7
Fathers	24	24	10	14	24	10	14	-	-	-
Subtotal	99	100	40	59	77	25	52	22	15	7
Study III										
Mothers										
White	53	76	27	26	29	14	15	24	13	11
Black	17	24	8	9	9	5	4	8	3	5
Subtotal	70	100	35	35	38	19	19	32	16	16
Total Parents (All Studies)										
Mothers	199	79	103	96	125	58	67	74	45	29
Fathers	54	21	28	26	54	28	26	-	-	-
Subtotal	253	100	131	122	179	86	93	74	45	29

Number of parents in family, and type of case

with their husbands. Of these 58% were separated, 21.5% divorced, 13.5% widowed, and 7% had never married. Some of the mothers who were separated had been separated for a long time while others were recent separations. In some instances the recent separations contributed to the mothers' need for psychiatric care. The model length of separation was a year longer in the urban group than in the suburban group. Black mothers had a longer period of separation of 5 years or over than white mothers.

In one-seventh of all families separated, parents had been separated for less than 1 month and in most of these there was evidence that the patients' hospitalizations or emergency visits followed crises brought on by the factors which contributed to the separation, such as husband's interests in other women, in-law difficulties, marital problems, or physical abuse. In a few families additional separations occurred during the study year for similar reasons and because the patient was readmitted to the hospital. Some parents were reunited during the study year. This occurred in 12 of the 54 families in Studies II and III. It is possible that the efforts of the social workers in the demonstrations contributed to these reunions since half of these were in the demonstration cases.

About the same proportion of ill mothers as ill fathers had had a prior marriage (12 and 13%). The distributions were similar also for white and black mothers. Of the 24 ill fathers all but 5 returned home from the hospital. Of the 5 who did not return, 2 died, 1 was divorced, 1 separated, and 1 was deserted by his wife who took the children with her.

Education

Ill mothers who had completed high school showed interesting comparisons with the 1960 figures for the Metropolitan Area. 54% of women in the Area completed high school as compared with 39% of mothers in Study I which included several industrial towns; 59% in

Study II which included more suburban and affluent areas; and 34% of white mothers in Study III, the City of Boston area. Black mothers in Study III had the lowest percentage, 29.5%, of high school education. On the whole, in Study III, the ill mothers attained a lower level of education than did women in the Metropolitan Area.

There are less apparent differences in the educational attainment of the ill fathers as compared with males in the Metropolitan Area. A smaller proportion of ill fathers received less than a seventh-grade education or failed to go beyond high school. Almost twice as many fathers in Study I failed to reach the tenth grade as in Study II. However, the numbers of fathers are small and the number of unknowns too great to draw sound comparisons between the sexes.

Religion

Of the 199 ill mothers, all but 12 gave a religious preference or admitted to no religion. Catholicism was the choice of 64% of mothers and 57% of ill fathers. This proportion of Catholic mothers was greater than the proportion of Catholics in the Metropolitan Area and in the City of Boston. Conversely the proportion of Protestant fathers was greater than the proportion of Protestant fathers in Boston and about the same proportion as that in the Metropolitan Area. The proportion of Jewish parents in these studies was considerably less than the proportion of Jews in the population of Boston or the Metropolitan Area. There were more Jewish mothers (10) in the studies than Jewish fathers (1). A larger proportion of black mothers in the studies were Protestant than the proportion in either the City of Boston or the Metropolitan Area.

Annual Income

The greater proportion of families with higher incomes lived in the small cities and suburban areas (Study II); the next highest in the industrial towns and their surroundings (Study I), while the smallest proportion was in the City of Boston (Study III). The high income levels in Study II reflected the inclusion in the study of an affluent city in which half of the families had incomes of over $1,250 per person per year.

There was a striking difference between the two-parent and one-parent families. Among the two-parent families in all three studies there was a considerable proportion living on small incomes or receiving public assistance. This proportion was greater when the father was the patient; thus the fathers' illness seriously affected the families' income. The proportion of white two-parent families in the Boston Study receiving public assistance was considerably greater than the proportion in Studies I and II.

One-parent families had a much higher proportion of low incomes ($750 per person per year) and of those receiving public assistance. In the city study the proportion of black families receiving public assistance was higher than the proportion of white families receiving public assistance. This was twice greater in the two-parent black families and 20% greater in the one-parent black families. Of the 8 one-parent black families, 7 were receiving public assistance.

Occupation and Employment Status

The modal occupation of all fathers including the ill fathers was operative or laborer. This was particularly marked in black families in Study III and ill fathers in Study II. A larger proportion of husbands of ill mothers was in the upper three occupational levels (47%) as compared with ill fathers (37%).

Few mothers (14%) were employed at the time of or immediately prior to their hospitalization or emergency care. This ranged from 20% in Study I, 13% in Study II, and 9% in Study III, showing that mothers in the city study tended to work less than mothers in the suburban studies. This relates to the higher proportion of families on public assistance in the urban study. Of the 27 ill mothers who worked, 11 were employed in a clerical or sales capacity, 3 each as nurses, nurses aids, or in factory work and the others in several types of employment. Over half of the mothers worked full-time and during the daytime.

When the fathers were ill the proportion of mothers who worked was considerably greater (47% in Study I and 33% in Study II) than when the mothers were ill (14%). Most of them, too, worked full-time during the daytime mostly in clerical or saleswork or in factories. Thus almost half of the mothers supported their families when the fathers became ill.

The proportion of husbands of ill mothers who were unemployed was greater in the city study than in the suburban studies. Also more of those husbands in the city study who were employed had held their jobs for less than 5 years and less than in the suburban study (24% of white husbands and 11% of black husbands in the city as compared with 58% of white husbands in the suburbs). The proportion of ill fathers who had held their jobs for 5 years or longer was less than the proportion of husbands of ill mothers (25% as compared with 58%) who held their jobs for 5 years or longer, indicating the effects of mental illness on job stability.

The black fathers, although small in number, had the highest proportion without employment at intake (44%) and the lowest with regular employment (56%).

Geographic Mobility

The data regarding mobility within the 5 years prior to the studies was available only for Study III and for some families in Study II. Of these 169 families over half (61%) had moved at least once. There had been more moving of families in the urban study, both white and black, than of families in the suburban study. In both studies one-parent families moved more than did two-parent families. Many more black one-parent families moved than did one-parent white families. In the suburban study there was more moving of families with ill fathers than with ill mothers.

Housing

About half of all the families (51%) rented their homes. The proportion of those families who owned their own homes was three times greater in Studies I and II than in Study III, reflecting the suburban factor in the first two studies. The proportion of two-parent families with ill mothers who owned their own homes was considerably greater than that of one-parent families or of families with ill fathers. A few families had no home of their own. These were mostly one-parent families who lived with relatives. Some homes of one-parent families were given up when the mothers became ill and were hospitalized and in only one of these families had the home been reestablished by the end of the study year.

Overcrowding was more frequently reported among one-parent than two-parent families (23% of one-parent families in Study II and 50% in Study III). Children in these families usually slept several to a room, or on couches, or sometimes shared beds. Parents and children, in some cases, shared the same room and occasionally the same bed.

Poor housekeeping resulting in dirty or filthy conditions was found in 9% of the homes in Study II when the mother was the ill parent and in considerably more of those in Study III (23%). There were fewer such conditions when the father was the ill parent. A small number of families had inadequate household furnishings.

In Study III a third of the families lived in deteriorating or slum neighborhoods; almost a fourth in three-family houses (22%) and somewhat less than a third in public housing developments (27%). A simple accounting of the types of dwellings or of a few of the living conditions, however, does not make clear the distressful conditions under which many of the Study III families lived. The following report by a research interviewer graphically portrays the conditions which were found in multiple family or tenement houses and in the housing developments.

The areas were blighted and ugly, and the tenement houses, the entrances, halls, and apartments were in many instances really unfit for human habitation. Entrance halls were dark and dirty with broken steps and railings, no electric lighting, no doorbells, no mailboxes, etc. In many apartments the paper was peeling off the walls, the floors were uncovered and grimy, the grit and decay were everywhere. Unfortunately, the housing projects were not much better. Even in the relatively newer ones hallways were littered with garbage and refuse, halls were unpainted, windows broken, the whole project bleak, unattractive, and uninviting.

For example, Mrs. E., diagnosed as an hysterical personality, lived with seven small children on the top floor of an old tenement. There was dirt everywhere; the apartment reeked of urine and vomitus, a result of poor housing and poor housekeeping.

The H. family, numbering five children and two adults, occupied three rooms on the fifth floor of a tenement block. The thirteen-year-old daughter slept in what was previously the pantry, a room so small that only one person could be in it at a time. Four boys, aged sixteen five, three, and two years, occupied one small narrow bedroom, and the parents slept in the back part of the living room. Although Mrs. H. tried hard to keep this house clean and neat, and largely succeeded, the overcrowding was an intolerable burden.

The C. family occupied the first floor of a frame dwelling which was so old and so decrepit it was hard to tell what kept it together. The furnishings were also old, inadequate, and falling apart, and Mrs. C. appeared to be a very poor housekeeper. She did not even seem aware of how inadequate her housing was.

Mrs. H. occupied an apartment which was so bad that the building had been condemned and she soon had to move. A poor housekeeper by nature, she was totally unable to cope with household tasks when feeling depressed. . . .

In many households there were not beds enough to go around, and often three or more children slept in one bed. Mrs. R. had beds enough but no mattresses. Little children were growing up in bleak, dirty, ugly, inadequate surroundings. In one household a mother on public assistance said she did not have enough money to buy the equipment, such as soap powder, to keep her house clean.

Pregnancies of Mothers

Information concerning the number of pregnancies of ill mothers and their outcomes was gathered by the research interviewers in all three studies (Table 2). In Study III it was supplemented by data obtained from the pediatrician among 56 of the 70 families in which he examined the children. The mean number of pregnancies was generally smaller (except in Study I) among one-parent families as would be expected. Two-parent families had more pregnancies in Study III than in the other two studies. Black mothers had the highest number. For one-parent families the mean is lowest in Study II, but is higher among both white and black families in Study III than in either of the earlier studies.

It is possible that the greater number of pregnancies in Study III reflects the supplementary information obtained from the pediatric histories. However, it also reflects fertility differentials in a general population associated with poverty and/or race.

The proportion of known pregnancies which ended in fetal deaths in the total was 12%. However, this is exceeded by both the black mothers (24%) in Study III and white two-parent mothers (14.5%) in Study II. Underreporting may account for the low fetal death rates in Study I.

THE ILL PARENTS

Several factors may contribute to the kind and severity of risks created for children when a parent is mentally ill: (1) whether the mother or father is the mentally ill parent; (2) the diagnosis of the ill parent (whether psychotic, psychoneurotic, or personality defect); (3) the age of the children at the onset of the parent's illness; (4) the need

TABLE 2
Number of reported pregnancies of ill mothers

Number of Pregnancies	Total mothers (N = 199)	I		II		III White		III Black	
		Two (N = 34)	One (N = 20)	Two (N = 53)	One (N = 22)	Two (N = 29)	One (N = 24)	Two (N = 9)	One (N = 8)
1-2	30.5%	38%	35%	37%	34%	17%	25%	22%	0%
3-4	37.5	53	45	37	36	34	33	11	12.5
5-6	16	6	15	17	19	21	25	0	25
7 or more	11.5	3	5	7	10	14	12.5	67	25
Unknown	4.5	0	0	1	2	14	4	0	37.5
Total	748	101	68	193	63	131	94	62	36
Mean	3.8	3	3.4	3.6	2.9	4.5	3.9	6.9	4.5

Study, race, and number of parents

for hospitalization of the parent; and (5) the length of hospitalization or recurrent readmissions. These factors may affect the impact on children of distress and disruption in the home, or the children's involvement in the illness of the parent. Other factors also may contribute, such as the economic or social status of the family, the accessibility of mental health resources, and the ability or the motivation of the patient to utilize resources. The most pervasive factors are the number of parents in the family and whether the ill parent is a father or a mother. The parental status of the family was a major variable, therefore, in the examination and description of the physical care and living arrangements of the children. One would expect that mental illness and hospitalization of a mother would result in more disruption in the care of the children that when a father was hospitalized. One would also expect that when the only parent in a family is the mother her hospitalization would create the greatest risk to the care of the children since then the children are without any parent in the home to care for them.

Presenting Problems—Studies I and II

In reviewing the literature there were no guides in establishing categories for the reasons or chief complaints or presenting problems. The patients' hospital records and the research schedules in Studies I and II showed that the chief complaints or presenting problems were frequently concerned with the children of these ill parents. In some cases presenting problems were given as frank, serious statements of highly suspicious or hostile involvement of the ill parent which would affect the well-being of children. Other statements indicated serious or overconcern with one or all of the children, often because of an illness or difficulty of a child, or because the mother was unable to carry out her usual and expected responsibilities for the children. The presenting problems were also related to other social or situational difficulties such as marital conflict, problems of housing, neighbors, or employment in addition to psychiatric or emotional complaints of affective disorders and delusional or hallucinatory experiences.

Because the ill parents in Studies I and II were hospitalized and those in Study III were infrequently hospitalized after their emergency visits, it might be expected that the presenting problems of patients in the three studies would be different. There is no substantiating data in the literature, however, to indicate that patients seen in psychiatric emergency services of general hospitals are "different," or have "different" presenting problems, either in substance or degree from those patients seen in state mental hospitals. This was true in these studies, also. Although the presenting problems of the mentally ill parents, whether hospitalized or not, contained frank reference to difficulties with their children, no systematic evaluation was made of the distrubance in the parental role or the extent of the distress or involvement of the children.

The presenting problems were those problems most frequently reported by the patient or relatives (Table 3). The problems were those related to children or to emotional or psychotic symptoms. Those presenting problems related to children were: (1) abuse, neglect, fear of harming; (2) worry about a child; (3) parent-child conflict; (4) inability to cope; and (5) pregnancy or birth.

Even though there was no systematic approach in the open-ended interview which specifically associated the parents' presenting problems with an impact on or involvement with the children, more than half of the parents (59%), and particulary the mothers (62%), presented their problems as directly related to their children or their own adequacy as parents. The proportions of mothers who reported child-related difficulties was 34% in Study I, 44% in Study II, and 46% in Study III, showing a greater proportion in the urban study. The extent of the difficulties for children cannot be fully appreciated unless the traditional emphasis on patient-oriented care and treatment is

TABLE 3
Types of presenting problems reported by 225 mentally ill patients
on the initial research interview

Type of Problem	Total mentally ill patients (N = 225) (a)	Ill parent and study				
		Mother			Father	
		I (N = 38)	II (N = 75)	III (N = 70)	I (N = 18)	II (N = 24)
Related to children						
Abuse, neglect, fear of harming	11%	21%	9%	9%	11%	4%
Worry about child	16	11	16	24	0	8
Parent-child conflict	6	8	4	12	0	0
Inability to cope	14	21	21	10	—	—
Pregnancy or birth	8	8	9	10	—	—
Total with a child related problem	37	34	44	46	11	13
Related to emotional or psychotic symptoms						
Delusions or hallucinations	24	33	32	12	28	17
Suicidal attempts, gestures or impulses	18	21	27	12	6	17
Other affective or somatic symptoms	55	53	53	66	45	42
Total with a symptom related problem	73	84	87	60	61	58
Total Study patients	253	54	75	70	30	24

(a) Columns do not add to 100% since some patients reported more than one type and others reported none.

broadened to include the knowledge of the patient as a parent and the implications of mental illness for the children. In those instances where a mother or family reported child-related problems, the question of the risk to the children and their usual care was well documented. Examples of such were: "I'm afraid I'm going to hurt my little children; two months ago I lost all interest in them and I feel guilty about it, but there's nothing I can do about it." or "I have a guilty feeling about my eight-year-old boy; he was born a year before I was married. Just before I came to the hospital I began thinking about it a lot and then I yelled to him the other day that he was illegitimate. He's cried ever since." or "I think my fifteen-year-old girl is pregnant and I'm worried about the poor report card she just brought home."

It is interesting, but not surprising, to note that the mothers reported these kinds of problems in substantially higher proportions than did the hospitalized fathers. The proportions for each of the five types of problems related to children reflect only those statements that were presented by the patients or families as reasons for the hospital admission or contact (not an evaluation or interpretation of the problems by the study staff). Further questions on the research interview relating to these problems of children showed them to be grossly underreported by patients and families. If a systematic inquiry about the children were made at the first psychiatric examination, it is expected that patients and families would indicate more difficulties in relation to the children.

An example of a presenting problem reported by the family of a 45-year-old, twice married mother indicated that about 3 weeks prior to her admission she felt "nervous." Although data regarding the children is seldom reported in the hospital record, in this instance the record did state that the patient's present difficulties started 7 years before, shortly after her second marriage, mostly with tension and aggravations between her and her three stepchildren. The oldest child, then 15 years of age, soon left home to live with his maternal grandmother because the patient had a violent temper and felt persecuted by her stepchildren. She had also chased the boy around the yard with a knife. In the past few years the patient had a habit of leaving the home frequently (about 20 to 25 times) after she and the children had disagreements, and of staying away for weeks at a time. When she returned home from her separations, she was very kind and loving to the children for about 2 weeks and would then revert to her agitated state, throwing dishes and other things at them. Prior to this, her first mental hospital admission, it was reported that she chased the two girls, aged 15 and 13 years, around the house with a knife and the hose of a vacuum cleaner. This patient was diagnosed as having a psychoneurotic reaction, mixed type, and was discharged home after 30 days' hospitalization.

Further data from the research interview disclosed that 5 years before this mother, upon her husband's insistance, had discussed her problems with their clergyman who had helped to arrange treatment with a private psychiatrist. After 5 weeks she refused any further appointments, and ever since had expressed great dislike for her minister. The research interview with the father further disclosed that 2 years prior to her admission the father had sent the older girl to the Society for the Prevention of Cruelty to Children to report his wife because she had just beat the girl. "I had hoped they would talk to my wife, but they didn't do much to help." In the 6-month research interview when the patient had been at home for 5 months, the father further reported, "Both girls stay in their rooms every night because their mother doesn't want them to visit with their friends and won't let anyone come to the house. She's so jealous of me, and the girls, too. I don't know if she's sick or if it's just her way." This mother had had no contact with any community agency following her hospital discharge. The presenting problem of nervousness, as well as the indications in her hospital record of chasing the children with a knife, apparently were not considered as possible risks to her children. The patient reported her hospital experience as helpful in that she "felt fine" while there and "I gained weight and enjoyed working in the kitchen."

The presenting problems related to emotional or psychotic symptoms were reported. These were: (1) delusions or hallucinations; (2) suicidal attempts, gestures, or impulses; and (3) other affective or somatic symptoms. The highest proportion of patients had affective or somatic complaints. Some patients presented problems of these types as well as child-related problems.

An example of a patient whose presenting problems, according to the hospital record, included only emotional or psychiatric symptoms, was that of a 36-year-old, three times married mother of two children, one of whom was living at home. The mother stated her problems both to the hospital and the research interviewer: "I began to feel depressed again and stayed in bed for about a month before I went to the hospital." This mother had had her third mental hospital admission 5 months previously. A diagnosis of psychoneurotic reaction, anxiety and depression (sociopathic traits), and psychophysiological respiratory disturbance had been consistent in all three hospitalizations even though they were in different hospitals. In addition to her three mental hospitalizations, she had had in the past 6 years as many as nine admissions to general hospitals because of asthma. Her 8-year-old child had been separated from her mother because of the mother's illness twelve times in the previous 6 years. In the research interview the mother reported that this 8-year-old girl was tall for her age, but weighed only 60 pounds. "She cries easily and gets almost hysterical. When she gets excited or people visit the home, she invariably vomits and has been doing this since the age of 2 years. She had to be carried bodily to school when I had my first mental hospitalization nearly 3 years ago, and she would vomit in school." The parents stated they had never thought of seeking any help from any community resource, but had taken her to a local physician who told them she might have had pinworms. During the current hospitalization her grandmother cared for her in the child's home. There was difficulty because the grandmother was "overstrict and didn't understand our child." The parents had told their child that this hospitalization was for the mother's asthma. The child's question to her father about the hospitalization was, "Is it catching—will I get it?" This child had many other serious disturbances in relation to her mother's hospitalizations and illnesses which were recounted during the research interview. The hospital record gave only slight reference to the child's situation stating, "Patient's mother is in the home evidently caring for her 8-year-old girl."

In the study interviews there were many clues to the probable risks to children due to parents' mental illness and hospitalizations. Difficulties in living arrangements and ordinary care of the children created hazards for children of varying degree. This was reflected in such statements as: "I haven't been able to sleep for a week"; "I'm afraid I'm going to kill my child"; "I'm afraid my son is going to lose his arms and his legs, his vision and his mind—all because of my special powers"; "I'm nervous and upset for no reason at all"; or the father who reported that all his children were "fine," when this was in fact a denial of serious problems with his children.

In these presenting problems it would seem imperative that the hospital examine the situation of the children whether they are still at home or elsewhere. This would be especially advisable where a mother had made a suicidal attempt or gesture. In these studies almost a third of the mothers (30%) presented problems of this nature. An example of the impact on children is one 20-year-old, divorced mother of two children aged 2 and 1 years, who was 2 months pregnant at the time of her admission. She had made a suicidal attempt by pill ingestion and was found comatose by her ex-husband. The mother-in-law, who was temporarily caring for the children until their fosterhome placement was arranged, reported to the research interviewer that the children were wandering half naked in and out of the house, and were taken in by neighbors until the police went to hospitalize the patient. The mother's statement in reference to her suicidal attempt was, "I wanted to end my life because I couldn't care for my children." Another young, divorced mother of two children, aged 2 years and 9 months, stated, "I couldn't go on caring for my children, so I put them to bed for their naps and then went into the bathroom and slashed my wrists." In at least two families the mothers tried to include the children in their suicidal attempt by gas; in other instances the children were the first to come upon the attempted suicide. Certainly in this type of situational stress the presenting problem requires a systematic evaluation of possible risks to the children's physical and emotional health.

The proportions of presenting problems shown for Studies I and II differed somewhat from Study III. Sixty percent of the mothers in Study III reported emotional or psychiatric difficulties, as opposed to 84 and 87% in Studies I and II. This was to be expected since mothers in Studies I and II were hospitalized. The subcategories of delusional or hallucinatory symptoms were somewhat less in Study III than Studies I and II, and other affective symptoms or somatic complaints were only slightly higher (66 vs. 53%).

Presenting Problems—Study III

The presenting problems in Study III were taken from two sources: (1) the psychiatric record which reported the mother's difficulties when she came, usually in crisis, to the emergency service; and (2) the research interview, which usually occurred in the patient's home shortly following her emergency visit. At the time of the mother's emergency visit, the problems reported by the psychiatrist in the emergency record contained a higher proportion of emotional and psychiatric difficulties and a lesser proportion of social and environmental difficulties, including child-related problems. Conversely, at the time of the research interviewers' contacts with the mothers in the homes, the presenting problems contained a higher proportion of social and environmental difficulties and a lesser proportion of emotional and psychiatric difficulties.

In the presenting problems of emotional or psychiatric symptoms, 77% of the mothers reported presenting problems of this nature in the research interviews, as opposed to 91% at the emergency service contact. The affective and somatic difficulties were reported by 66% of the mothers within the research interview and 81% in the emergency visit contact. Essentially no difference was noted in the subcategory of delusional or hallucinatory complaints; 13% reported symptoms of this nature in the research interview, as opposed to 20% in the emergency visit.

In the presenting problems related to the social and environmental difficulties which included problems related to children, there was a higher proportion reported in the research interview than in the emergency record. These differences may be accounted for by at least three reasons: (1) The patients undoubtedly feel it appropriate and beneficial to present emotional and psychiatric difficulties to a psychiatrist in a hospital setting to a far greater degree than to a social worker in a home visit. Conversely, they feel it more appropriate and beneficial to present difficulties relating to their children, their marital conflicts, other relationships, and their financial situation to a social worker seeing them in their own home than to a psychiatrist in a hospital. (2) The time differential itself may have been a reason why patients reported their problems in a different perspective; they may have tended to deny or de-emphasize the emotional or psychiatric component within their problems or they may have lost some of the "crisis" concerns about their emotional or psychiatric problems and thereby emphasized their social or environmental problems which may not have been as threatening for them. (3) The psychiatrist in recording the interview may have placed more emphasis on the emotional or psychiatric difficulties than on the social and environmental problems.

These reasons, however, would not necessarily indicate that the problems had changed. For example, complaints of housing or finances would not change in such a short time, yet only 20% of the patients were stated to have such problems in the emergency report in contrast to 39% in the research interview report.

In both the emergency record and the research interview, marital difficulties were reported by approximately one-third of the mothers. The marital conflicts ranged from those of serious long-standing disrupting circumstances, particularly as they related to the situation of the children. Marital conflicts were reported by both one- and two-parent families. In a few instances an apparent precipitating cause of the patients' emergency visits were recent separations of husbands. Some husbands left the home very shortly after the emergency visit. For example, a 21-year-old mother of two children, aged 2 years and 13 months, came to the emergency service stating, "I want help for my husband." Two nights prior to her visit he had attempted to strangle her, and she was worried that he would try it again. She was also worried about his health and the fact that he had had a recent psychiatric outpatient department appointment which he had refused to keep. The hospital record further stated that this patient was "depressed and weepy, but abruptly pulled herself together and walked out when a possible solution was suggested." The husband had been separated from the family 1 month prior to the patient's emergency visit, had returned to the home 2 days prior to visit at which time he tried to strangle her, and then 2 days after her emergency visit when the research interviewer visited, he had left the home again.

Another patient, a 20-year-old mother of three children, aged 4 years, 1 year, and 7 months, was brought to the emergency service by ambulance since her husband hit her on the back of her neck, knocking her unconsicious. He had arranged for his wife's hospital visit after phoning his mother who advised him to call an ambulance. The presenting problem given by this patient was that she and her husband fought constantly, a fact which he corroborated when he accompanied the patient to the hospital. He accused her of infidelity, and she accused him of being a poor provider and abusing her. She further stated she was very upset "this morning because the children were dirty." She had not been able to sleep for some time, had no appetite, and had lost about twenty pounds in the last 2 months. Her husband was scheduled for an appointment in the alcoholic clinic of the hospital 2 days following her visit which he did not keep. In addition to this, he left home following his wife's emergency visit, a fact which was not determined until the time of the research interview when the patient was located in her mother's home.

The complaints of marital conflicts often included statements which indicated long-standing and serious effects of disruptions in child care, such as that of a 40-year-old mother of four children who stated her husband had beaten her for 20 years and had kept her "hostage" much of the time. There was no record of this woman ever seeking help for her marital situation from any community resource prior to this emergency visit. Another 38-year-old mother of four children came to the emergency service because she "had a fight last night with my husband, and I'm afraid I might kill him with a knife—he's cheating on me. When I walked out on my children this morning, I didn't know what to do or where to go and thought I might throw myself in front of a car." Another mother of three children—17, 13, and 9 years—came to the emergency service with the complaint of 18 years of marital difficulties, and was given the diagnosis of neurotic depression with an hysterical attempt at suicide to manipulate her husband and children. The patient accused her husband of staying out late at night and of alienating their 17-year-old daughter against her. The children were constantly badgered between the two parents to take sides, and the emergency visit was precipitated by the 17-year-old "squealing" to her father about punishment the patient was giving the 13-year-old. The patient took an overdose of pills in retaliation. The record further

TABLE 4
Duration of presenting problems among 235 study patients

	Ill parent, study, and type of case									
	Mother						Father			
	Study I						Study I			
Duration	Total patients (N = 253)	Demonstra-tion (N = 38)	Control (N = 16)	Study II (N = 75)	Study III (N = 70)		Demonstra-tion (N = 18)	Control (N = 12)		Study II (N = 24)
Less than 6 months	56%	66%	63%	57.5%	47%		50%	58%		58%
6 months to 1 year 11 months	18	13	25	17.5	24		17	8.5		13
2 to 4 years 11 months	10	2.5	0	10.5	11.5		5.5	8.5		25
5 years and over	7	8	6	5	6		22	8.5		0
Unknown	9	10.5	6	9.5	11.5		5.5	16.5		4

stated that the 9-year-old boy seemed to be taking "the brunt" of the marital conflict and recently had had contact with a child guidance center for a speech impediment and rather serious relationship difficulties. In this family the children had not been separated but long-standing marital conflicts had caused serious disruptions in the home and the care of the children. The disruptions in the lives of children caused both by periodic separations and by constant marital disturbances in the home are reality problems which are sadly compounded by mental and emotional illnesses.

There have been large increases in the number of people seeking care in emergency services, many of which were due to problems within social and family-life stress situations which may or may not be true psychiatric crises or emergencies. The above situations illustrated presenting problems which included those stress factors within marital relationships, difficulties in child rearing and parent-child relations, conflicts derived from unwanted pregnancies or childbirth, economic difficulties, and many others that may or may not be superimposed upon an existing psychiatric component. What is clear from examining these presenting problems of social and psychiatric symptomatologies is their serious impact on children.

Duration of Presenting Problems

The duration of presenting problems prior to the patient's hospitalization or emergency visit was found to be less than 1 week's time in 10% of the patients (Table 4). About the same proportion felt their presenting problems had existed for 5 years or more. In Study I there was little difference between mental hospital patients and sanatoria patients in the length of their complaints prior to hospital admission. In the three studies the ill fathers had slightly shorter durations of symptoms than the mothers. An unexpected finding was the proportion of patients whose symptoms had existed for 6 months or more before they sought treatment, a range from 23.5% to as high as 44% in the three studies. Therefore disruptive or distressful situations for children had existed in the home for a considerable length of time.

Prior Mental Hospitalizations

Almost half (45%) of all mentally ill mothers had had prior admissions to a mental hospital. This proportion was greater for the hospitalized mothers in Studies I and II than for the emergency patients, but a third of the emergency patients had been in a mental hospital before. Parents from two-parent families had more prior hospitalizations than from one-parent families except in Study I where ill mothers in one-parent families had more prior hospitalizations. Mothers of one-parent families with fewer prior mental hospital admissions did not have different mental diagnoses. For example in Study II of the mothers with psychotic diagnoses there was no appreciable difference between mothers in families of one or two parents. Just over two-thirds of all psychotic mothers had had prior admissions, but 75% of the mothers in two-parent families had had prior admissions as compared with 50% of the mothers in one-parent families. In other diagnostic categories the trends were consistently in the same direction.

The proportions of mentally ill fathers with prior admissions were 61% in Study I and 67% in Study II. These proportions were less than the proportions for mothers in two-parent families but higher than those for mothers in one-parent families. These differences between the readmissions of mothers in one- and two-parent families suggest that mothers in one-parent families may defer seeking medical care fearing that hospitalization would be advised, thus leaving their children without a parent to care for them.

Diagnoses of Ill Parents

As would be expected, Studies I and II with hospitalized parents had higher proportions of parents with psychotic diagnoses (45 and 59% for mothers) than Study III mothers (18%) seen in the emergency service. On the other hand, Studies I and II had lower proportions of mothers diagnosed as psychoneurotic (34 and 21%) than Study III mothers (53%) in the emergency services. In Study III only a few mothers were hospitalized as a result of the emergency visit.

There was very little difference in the proportions of mothers in one-parent and two-parent families with diagnoses of psychosis and psychoneurosis. With a diagnosis of personality disorders there was a slightly higher proportion of mothers in Study III than Studies I and II. The number of mothers with diagnoses of personality disorders was relatively small but there was a slightly greater tendency for the mothers of one-parent families to be so diagnosed.

In the total group of seventy mothers in Study III, seventeen (24%) were black, nine of whom were mothers in two-parent families and eight were of one-parent families. When the diagnostic categories in Study III were controlled for race, six (46%) of the thirteen mothers diagnosed as psychotic were black, more than twice the proportion of white mothers so diagnosed in Study III. Five (14%) of the thirty-seven mothers with psychoneurosis were black or three times less than the proportion for white mothers in Study III. Six (32%) of the nineteen mothers with personality disorders were black, about the same proportion as for white patients. The number of black patients, however, was too small to draw any reliable conclusions.

The proportions of the fathers in the different diagnostic categories were not comparable between Studies I and II because fathers with a diagnosis of alcoholism were not included in Study II. Also the number of fathers was too small from which to draw comparisons.

Length of Hospitalization

There was no consistent trend in the length of hospitalizations of ill parents to differentiate the mothers from one-parent families from those in two-parent families. Also there were no differences in length of hospitalization between Studies I and II for mentally ill parents. In Study III only seven mothers were hospitalized directly after the emergency visit; eighteen other mothers were admitted to a mental hospital during the study year. There was an interesting difference between Studies I and II and Study III in relation to the length of hospitalization. In Studies I and II the majority of the mothers had up to 3 months of hospital care while in Study III, of those hospitalized, the majority remained only 1 month or less and no mother had over 3 months hospitalization. In Study III mothers of two-parent families stayed in the hospital a longer time than mothers of one-parent families.

Of the nine mothers of one-parent families in Study III, four were released with less than 2 weeks care; three of these were rehospitalized (one mother was diagnosed as having personality disorder and two with psychoneurotic depressive reaction). Of the ten mothers of two-parent families, seven had hospitalizations of 2 weeks or less and of these, four were rehospitalized (three were diagnosed as having personality disorders and one was psychotic). Therefore, of these eleven mothers with hospital care of 2 weeks or less, at least one-half were readmitted within short periods of time and all within a year.

In Study I, six (11%) of the thirty-eight mentally ill mothers were readmitted to the mental hospital within the 6 month study period as were four (22%) of the mentally ill fathers. No tuberculous patients were readmitted since most of them were still in the hospital. In Study

II a somewhat larger proportion of patients from two-parent families than from one-parent families were readmitted. Fifteen (28%) of the fifty-three mentally ill mothers of two-parent families were readmitted as were four (18%) of the twenty-two mothers of one-parent families. Six (25%) of the twenty-four mentally ill fathers were readmitted during the study year. The numbers are small but in this study they indicate that the shorter the duration of hospitalization (2 weeks or less) the greater the tendency for readmission.

With mothers rehospitalized, repeated planning for the living arrangements of their children was necessary and children had to adjust and readjust to substitute caretakers. Children also showed concern and confusion as to the reasons for their mothers' behavior and rehospitalization. Mothers' comments indicate the distress experienced by children when mothers were sent away again: "Our 4-year-old cried constantly for 2 days when her mother went to the hospital"; "It's hard on everyone, but particularly the children"; "Disciplining the children seemed to be the big problem; they didn't know why their mother went away"; or "They put such hope in their mother's hospitalization—they thought she'd be all better when she came home."

Mental Hospitalization of Relatives

Approximately one-third of the relatives of these parents were reported to have had mental hospital care. Others were probably not included in the reports since some parents had had no contact with their relatives for some time. One relative reported that a 14-year-old boy had killed his father in trying to protect his mother during a marital argument. There were also four families in which the mothers and fathers were both hospitalized at the same time, three of them for mental illness. Other families had both parents hospitalized during the study year but not at the same time and not always for mental illness.

Some families called on mentally ill relatives to care for the children.

The research interviewers thought that some of these relatives caring for the children were as sick as the hospitalized mother.

Deaths

In Study I two hospitalized fathers died within the 6-month period of the study, both with the diagnosis of chronic brain syndrome associated with alcoholism. One was a 48-year-old father of two children and the other a 51-year-old father with one child. Both fathers had had prior mental hospitalizations. In Study II there were five mentally ill parents, three mothers and two fathers, who died within the study year. One 50-year-old mother of a 15-year-old child died of cancer. The second was a 39-year-old mother of six children who died from a drug sensitivity after 1 month's hospitalization. Her death was very upsetting to her children who had gone to the hospital to visit her. She became ill while they were taking her for a drive and by the time they had returned to the hospital she had died. Prior to her hospitalization, she had complained bitterly about the care of her children, stating that they gave her a nervous headache. During her hospitalization the children were being unsatisfactorily cared for by their 74-year-old paternal grandmother who was not able to manage the care of six children. Following the mother's death, the children were separated from their home, their father, and each other since they were sent to different relatives in another state. The third mother was 45 years old and had a 13-year-old son. She was hospitalized for 2 months and was diagnosed as psychotic depressive reaction. When she returned home, she was unable to concentrate and had little interest in anything at all, including her son. She constantly expressed fears that the neighbors had turned against her and her son. Four months after her hospital discharge, she committed suicide.

Of the two fathers who died, one was 39 years old with four children. He died of a brain tumor. The second father was 50 years old, had been "sickly" for many years, and died in the mental hospital of complications from a metabolic disorder. He had an 11-year-old daughter who was heartbroken at her father's death, since he spent much time with her at home between hospitalizations. His wife worked regularly and long hours to support the family and had very little time with their daughter. His death was reported to be a serious loss for the child.

These children, therefore, experienced the loss of a parent, first by hospitalization and then by death. The care, particularly of the younger children, was somewhat precarious during the hospitalizations of the parents and in most instances deteriorated after the parents' death when some homes were discontinued and children were scattered among relatives or in foster homes.

Summary

The ill parents in these studies were mostly middle-aged. They were equally divided between ill father, ill mothers in two-parent families, and ill mothers in one-parent families. More than three-fourths of the ill mothers were not living with the husbands, most of them for reasons of separation. The short periods of separation were related to the strains of mental illness. More ill mothers than ill fathers had less than a high school education and the black parents had the least education. There was a higher proportion of Catholics in the group than in the population of the area. The fathers and the black parents had a higher proportion of Protestants than the ill mothers. There were fewer Jews than the proportion in the population. In general the income was low except in the affluent city of Study II. In the City of Boston study, incomes were the lowest and in the one-parent families they were generally below the poverty level. Many of these families were receiving public assistance.

Unemployment and less steady employment was highest in the urban families, especially among the black families. The largest number of fathers were operatives or laborers. Sick fathers held jobs less long than husbands of ill mothers. Few mothers worked, especially in the urban study. When mothers did work they generally worked during the day and full-time.

There was a high rate of mobility, over half of the families having moved within the 5 years previous to the study. Black families and families with ill fathers moved more often than the other families. One-parent families moved more often than two-parent families. Three times more families in the suburban studies owned their own homes than families in the urban study. Over half of all families rented their homes. There were a few families who had no homes of their own and a few with homes given up due to the mothers' mental illness. Half of the families lived in overcrowded quarters. In the urban study a third lived in deteriorating or slum neighborhoods and a quarter had poor housekeeping. Deplorable conditions were common in the urban study.

The kinds and severity of risks to children because of the parent's mental illness varied according to which parent was ill, the diagnosis of the ill parent, the age of the children, the need for hospitalization, and the length and recurrence of hospital care. Over a third of the presenting problems were those related to children and two-thirds those related to emotional or psychotic symptoms of the ill parent. In the suburban studies over half of the patients had psychotic diagnoses while in the urban study over half had a diagnosis of psychoneurosis. The child-related problems were infrequently recorded in the hospital record even though many of them were of a serious nature. From a quarter to a half of all the patients had had symptoms of mental illness for 6 months or longer before going to the emergency service or the hospital. Stresses and strains on children had existed in these homes for a considerable length of time.

Almost half of the mentally ill mothers hospitalized had had one or more prior admissions to a mental hospital while a third of those in the emergency service had had prior mental hospital care. Only a few of the emergency patients were hospitalized from the emergency service.

Almost half of the patients remained in the hospital from 1 to 2 months. Those who left after 2 weeks or less had pressures from home responsibilities. Half of these patients were readmitted during the study year. Two to three times higher proportion of mothers in the urban study left the hospital within 1 month than in the suburban studies. One-third of the relatives of all the patients were reported to have been hospitalized for mental illness.

Potential risks created for children in these families are apparent.

5

Impact of Parental Illness on Children

Hospitalization of ill parents in the three studies caused many disturbances and disruptions in the normal activities of these families. The children were variously involved in the emotional disturbances occurring in their homes. With the mental illness of one parent and the emotional strain on the other, children were exposed to a wide range of upsetting experiences in their day-to-day existence. Some children were intimately involved in the bizarre symptomatologies of their parents while others were not aware of the parents' illness and experineced no apparent difficulties because of it.

The reporting of the experiences of the children was obtained from the initial research interviews. In Studies I and II these were usually held with the substitute child caretaker or the father in the case of a hospitalized mother. When fathers were hospitalized the mothers provided the data in the interviews. In Study III the mentally ill mothers were consistently interviewed. The description of the experiences or the extent of involvement of the children varied somewhat according to the repondents' relationship to the children and the extent to which the respondents were aware of the problems.

Number and Ages of Children

There were 652 children in these 253 families or a mean average of 2.7 children per family. Fifty-two percent were boys and 48% girls. Almost half of the children were under 6 years of age (42%) and almost a quarter under 3 years of age (23%). They were fairly evenly distributed among the three studies and the parent groups. The proportion of two-parent families with four or more children was most marked in Studies II and III in which the proportion was almost twice as great as that of the Metropolitan Area. The mean number of children in Study III in both one- and two-parent families was greater than that in the other studies.

In Study III of the one-parent families 10% of the white children and 33% of the black children were known or suspected of having been born out-of-wedlock. In two-parent families this was true of only one white and one black child. This data was not available for Studies I and II and is probably underestimated for Study III.

Effects of Parents' Illness on Children

Questions about the effects of the parents' illness on children were often threatening to the families. Mentally ill mothers occasionally assumed that the research interviewer was there to take the children away. This reaction was more prevalent among mothers who had questioned their own maternal adequacy.

The families' reports as to whether the symptomatology of the illness had an impact or made any difference to the children were simply divided into children being (1) upset, and (2) neglected or abused. Among the control families in Study I only six (38%) of the sixteen mothers hospitalized for tuberculosis reported their children were upset in relation to the illness. The families of ill fathers reported no impact of their illness on the children. No families with tuberculosis reported neglect or abuse of children. In this group of tuberculous patients the time available to prepare the children for the expected hospitalization of the parent was beneficial. Families were able to arrange their financial affairs, to obtain substitute child-care, and to explain the illness and thereby lessen the distress to children. On the other hand the children in families of mentally ill parents in all three studies were involved in their parents' symptomatology in a higher proportion of families and in different ways than in the families with tuberculosis. An example of children being upset was reported by Mr. H. who stated that his two children, aged 16 and 12 years, cried a lot because of their mother's actions. For 1 month prior to her admission the children realized she would have to return to the hospital again (she had had five prior hospitalizations in the past 9 years). She told them that the people upstairs were listening in to everything. Then she refused to have the children's friends come to the house. "She did all sorts of things to upset us all, like saying we had to move from our apartment because the neighbors were talking about her. She also went to a lawyer to get separate support and threatened to kick me out of the house. The children were very upset with all this. They cried a lot and were sad to see their mother getting sick again."

In another family, Mr. S. reported that his wife's reactions upset their 14-year-old girl. Mrs. S. had had as many as ten mental hospitalizations in the past 10 years and preceding each of her admissions, "she became violent and uncontrollable, went on wild shopping sprees, made nonsensical telephone calls, and smashed radios or anything else around the house. Just before she went to the hospital this time, she made a long distance telephone call to my eldest daughter in Kansas who is a freshman in college. My wife talked so irrationally it upset her, too. She cried so much that she is coming home and I'll have to try to calm her down. But it's my youngest girl who really got involved in my wife's antics. She tried to restrain her mother as best she could by hiding the radio and trying to keep her mother from using the telephone. It's a big experience for a child even if she has grown somewhat accustomed to it."

Other remarks by families in reporting that the children were "upset" included statements such as: "My two boys were terribly upset when their father started accusing me of going with other men. This wasn't like him and the boys didn't know what was what"; or, "My husband broke the children's toys and made them cry day after day until he went to the hospital"; or, "I don't know what this has been doing to my little girl (8 years old). I found her and three of her playmates peeking in the windows watching my wife's strange behavior. Then they all giggled and began to tease my girl and my wife." Several families reported their children were embarrassed by the parents' symptoms, while other families said the children "are getting used to the shade pulling, or the pan throwing, but it upsets them each time just the same."

There were a few families in which a child apparently mimicked or assumed symptoms of a parent. In one family the 18-year-old daughter would not eat any food her father had prepared. Her mother's symptoms had included paranoid ideation which centered on accusations that her husband was poisoning the food. Another, a 5-year-old girl gargled as her mother had done when she attempted suicide by ingestion of sleeping pills. In another family the 2-year-old boy drank fuel oil following his mother's suicide attempt by ingestion and had to have his stomach pumped.

Other children were reported to be abused by ill parents. For example, one 32-year-old mother of four children, aged 12, 8, 2 years, and 9 months, was reported by the family to hit and to bite the children. They felt her difficulties started after the birth of her youngest child when she tied the youngest child's leg to his crib since that was the only way she could keep him where she wanted him. In another family the 15-year-old child fled in terror when her mother threatened her with a knife. This child was also beaten on the head when she was sick in bed with a fever. Another mother 19 years old, had complained of feeling "funny" and prior to her emergency visit had beaten the 19-month-old baby because he wouldn't stop crying. The child's leg was broken and he was hospitalized.

Some children were reported to beg that the ill parent be

hospitalized. Others expressed relief when the parent was admitted. One mother reported that she felt her children were not involved in their father's illness but stated that they were more relaxed and slept better after he was hospitalized. He had frightened the children (ages 15 to 3 years) by his actions since he sat around the house all day and criticized everything the children did. He began to talk queerly and said "the birds were confusing things and inoculating things." The father had had four hospitalizations for mental illness and each time the mother had insisted that the children not be told that he was ill. At the time of this admission she told them that he had gone to a retreat house to rest. This upset and confused the children all the more.

Among those families that reported no involvement of the children in the illness of the parent there were indications from the data that this was not the case. For example, of the twenty-six mentally ill mothers in Study II in which no involvement of the children was reported, other statements indicated that the children in at least fifteen of these twenty-six families were involved in the illness. In thirteen of the fifteen families the mothers had complained of not being able to care for the children or to cope with them. Also in four of these fifteen families the mothers had made suicidal attempts and the children were present at these traumatic events. Among these twenty-six families there were fourteen (54%) in which all the children were 6 years of age or younger.

The involvement of the children in the symptomatology of the parents' illness, therefore, ranged from relatively minor, upsetting incidents related to transient events to those grave, traumatic experiences of serious impact. In the latter experiences the children showed confusion, bewilderment, fright, or sadness. Some received unprovoked beatings and in some instances frank abuse resulting in physical injuries. To determine the long-term effect of such experiences on the lives of these children would require an intensive study of the children over a longer period of time than these studies covered.

Psychosocial Difficulties of Children

The children's difficulties were separated into two general categories of behavioral difficulties and neurotic traits. They ranged from relatively minor or transient problems, such as nail-biting, to those of major or critical proportions such as serious delinquent acts. For example, a 12-year-old boy placed dynamite he had stolen under his house "to blow it up because of the awful things my father said about my mother."

The proportions of children in the three studies who were reported by the families to have difficulties were controlled for children of mentally ill mothers and mentally ill fathers (Table 5). Study I, in addition, was controlled for mentally hospitalized parents and parents hospitalized with tuberculosis. In Study I the proportion of children of mentally ill parents with difficulties is considerably higher than the proportion of children with tuberculous parents. The proportions of children with mentally ill fathers reported to have difficulties in Study I are much higher than those in Study II (59 vs. 38%). This difference may be due to the fact that mothers were usually the informants when fathers were ill. Also over one-half of the eighteen mentally ill fathers in Study I were diagnosed as having chronic brain syndrome due to alcoholism. Only four of the thirty-eight mentally ill mothers in Study I had a primary diagnosis of alcoholism. The proportions of children of mentally ill mothers who were reported to have difficulties are strikingly similar throughout the three studies.

More families reported that their children had neurotic traits than behavioral problems. The children of mentally ill fathers in Study I again had the highest proportion of neurotic traits. Among the children of mentally hospitalized mothers in Studies I and II similar proportions of neurotic traits and behavioral difficulties were reported. In Study III the proportion of neurotic traits was somewhat less than the proportion of behavioral difficulties.

TABLE 5
Children with behavioral or neurotic type difficulties

		Ill parent, study, and type of case						
		Mother				Father		
		Study I				Study I		
Difficulty	Total children (N = 652)	Demonstration (N = 85)	Control(a) (N = 43)	Study II (N = 188)	Study III (N = 215)	Demonstration (N = 41)	Control (a) (N = 25)	Study II (N = 55)
Reported	48%	47%	33%	53%	52%	59%	16%	38%
Not reported	52	53	67	47	48	41	84	62
Total difficulties reported	556	72	20	182	203	40	4	35
Behavioral	(186)	(19)	(5)	(57)	(90)	(6)	(0)	(9)
Neurotic traits	(370)	(53)	(15)	(125)	(113)	(34)	(4)	(26)
Total families	253	38	16	75	70	18	12	24

(a) Tuberculous patients.

TABLE 6
Types of difficulties reported among study children by age

	Total children (a) (N = 652)	Age (years)				
Type of difficulty		0-2 (N = 143)	3-5 (N = 122)	6-12 (N = 242)	13-17 (N = 126)	18-21 (N = 19) (b)
Behavioral						
Hard to manage	11%	8%	15%	12%	10%	0%
Temper tantrums	6	3.5	7	5	8	0
Excessively shy	7.5	1	4	10	11	10.5
Delinquent acts	4	0	3	3	9	5
Other	1	0	0	0	2	16
Neurotic traits						
Nail-biting	10	2	7	11	16	26
Enuresis	7	0	12	10	5	0
Eating difficulties	9	8	11	10	5	10.5
Sleeping difficulties	7	4	14	7	3	0
Headaches	2	0	0	2.5	6	5
Fears	7	1	4	5	3	0
"Nervous"	15	4	17	20	18	10.5
Other	1	0	3	7	0	5
None	52	77.5	48	39	49	63

(a) Columns do not add to 100% since any child may have had more than one type of difficulty.
(b) Study I only.

The proportions of children with specific types of problems in the categories of behavioral difficulties and neurotic traits are shown by age groups (Table 6). Over half (52%) of the 652 children were reported to have no difficulties; the age group 6-12 years had the smallest proportion without difficulties. There is reason to believe that underreporting was prevalent in all age groups and that further evaluation of the children would reveal more difficulties both in number and severity.

The highest proportion of children with difficulties (15%) was reported as being nervous. One 14-year-old child was described as having a "sick stomach when she is upset because of her mother's actions, and this is quite often." Two 9-year-old twins were both said to be high-strung and nervous. They both chewed their hair and one twin would not eat and cried a lot. In the 0-2 year age group, there were six (4%) children whose mothers or families felt they were nervous. One mother reported her 2-year-old child to be nervous, "mostly because of me, I guess; I never wanted her and I know I hit her whenever she whines because that drives me crazy. I think she's afraid of me, but she does things to bother me, too, like wetting on the floor on purpose." This child was also reported to be rebellious and hard to control. In the 3-5 year age group, 17% (21) of the children were so described; this proportion is essentially the same as in the groups 6-12 and 13-17 years.

Nail-biting was reported among 10% of the children, which was not a high proportion. However, some parents reported that their children "bite their nails something awful." One 14-year-old girl (control family) who "bites her fingernails 'til they bleed," also "bites her toenails and they become infected so she had to see a doctor." This child had had sexual advances made to her by her alcoholic father and was reported to be "going out with older boys and taking speed drives in their cars." Also, she was one of three children noted in behavioral difficulties under "other" because of suicidal gestures; she had taken an overdose of aspirin and was referred by her physician to a psychiatrist. A second child in the "other" category, a 15-year-old girl, slashed her wrists after a fight with her boy friend. This child (also in a control family) became illegitimately pregnant during the study year and left school to be married. Her younger sister, 12 years old, was forced to accompany the alcoholic mother to bars, and also became intoxicated. The third child in the "other" category, a 6-year-old, was suspended from school because she "tried to hang herself from a desk."

In relation to eating and sleeping there was a slight tendency for children of one-parent families to show greater proportions of difficulties. The proportion of children with no difficulties reported was less in one-parent families than in two-parent families in all the studies. When fathers were ill in Study I there was a higher proportion of children with difficulties in nail-biting and enuresis, while in Study II there was a higher proportion with sleeping problems and fears. This difference in type of problem may be due to the fact that 40% of the fathers in Study I were hospitalized for tuberculosis.

School

Almost two-thirds of all the children were in school. In Study I there was a higher proportion of children not in school than in the other studies because children 18-21 years, most of whom had been graduated from high school, were included in this study. A few of them were school dropouts under 18 years of age in all the studies. An example is that of a 6-year-old girl who was suspended from school because she was unmanageable. She was sent to an aunt in Florida because her 34-year-old mother, who had four other children (aged 16, 10, 5 years, and sixteen months), couldn't "stand her" and related her present fear of going insane, like her father, to have started when this child was born. She stated that she made a serious effort to abort her last pregnancy by taking pills, and said "these just burned out my whole bladder." The aunt in Florida returned the child to her mother after 2 days because she couldn't "stand her, either." Following this the child was sent to a grandmother in Oklahoma, but was returned home after a few months because they didn't get along. By the end of the study year, this child had been placed in a children's institution through the efforts of the demonstration social worker. One of the 16-year-old dropouts was a member of this same family. He had left school when he became 16 and went to work to help out at home. This boy worked for a time heating shellac in a shellac pit, but left home precipitously to join the Job Corps to get away from home and was sent to Texas. After 1 month, he became homesick, left the Job Corps, and returned home to a similar job as before. The father in the family was in and out of the home during the year (mostly out). At the time of the final interview the mother was again pregnant.

Another girl left school on her sixteenth birthday. Her mother had been forcibly removed from the home to a mental hospital because of extremely bizarre behavior, which included suicidal gestures as well as homicidal acts toward her children and her husband. During the study year this child got married to get out of the house.

A 16-year-old boy who dropped out of school had returned home from a correctional institution where he had been sent after killing his father who had attacked his mother during a wild fight. The boy had hoped to return to school but in spite of repeated efforts of the demonstration social worker he became a hero and a leader in a gang of delinquent boys who were also school dropouts.

Another 16-year-old boy was on probation at the time of his leaving school because he had hit a guard in a subway station. His mother complained about him, saying he was not working, drank a lot, and went with a bad group. He often stayed out late at night or did not go home for several nights and his mother did not know where he was or what he was doing. Subsequently he joined the Army.

Repeated Grades

Almost a quarter of the children had repeated grades in school. There was a slightly higher proportion of children in the families of mentally ill parents as opposed to the families with tuberculous parents. It was surprising that in Studies II and III the children of one-parent families had markedly fewer repeated grades than those of two-parent families. A higher proportion of children in black families in Study III repeated grades than did children in white families; this was more true of the children in two-parent black families than black children in one-parent families.

Academic Standing

The academic standing was reported by the schools in Studies II and III. There was a higher proportion of children in Study II who were reported by their teachers to be average students or at grade placement than in Study III which had a rather large proportion of children considered to be below grade placement by their teachers. This may be accounted for in part by a superior school system in one of the towns included in Study II. With only one exception there was a higher proportion of children of one-parent families in the above grade placement and at grade placement than in two-parent families and a lower proportion in below grade placement. One reason for this may be the absence of severe marital discord which was reported in one-half of the two-parent families.

Twenty-four children (22% of children in school) were in the above average academic group. Two negative factors were frequently identified within the home situations of these children: (1) serious or long-standing marital conflicts, and (2) difficulties in child care, such as disturbances in mother-child relations with poor or inconsistent child care. Two negative factors reported by the schools were: (1) behavioral difficulties in the school, and (2) problems related to absence or tardiness of a child.

In this group of above average academic standing there are other interesting differences between children of one- and two-parent families. The average age of the children was similar (8.4 and 8.3 years), but the children in one-parent families were advanced in grade level with the average grade being 3.6 (fourth grade) as compared with 2.9 (third grade) in the children of two-parent families. With these children of above average academic standing, problems in the family situations were often coexistent with the children's behavior problems in school.

Children in Two-Parent Families—Study III

In the two-parent group in Study III just over two-thirds of the nine children with above academic standing were subjected to serious marital conflicts within their homes. An example of the pervasive impact of marital conflict was that of an 8-year-old child whose 36-year-old mentally ill mother went to a psychiatric emergency service because of constant arguments with her husband. She felt that their marital conflicts were definitely affecting the children for they had become harder to manage. This mother of nine children from 14 to 2 years of age further reported that her husband drank too much, resulting in many arguments which bothered the children. Their father's drinking also embarrassed them in front of their friends; the younger children were at home to see and hear the commotion while the older children were often at the homes of relatives or friends. She further said: "My husband hits me and I throw things at him. The children are tense and nervous and even hard to control. I'm afraid I'll do something to their father. We've had the police come to the house because of the fighting." The school reports on the 8-year-old child in this family indicated she was above average academically, quite an intelligent child but tended to be withdrawn and needed much praise to prevent withdrawal. Beyond this she showed no problems. The teacher did not report any home difficulties which might have been bothering the child. Interestingly the school reports on the other children in this family, not in the above average group, indicated frequent absences which affected their school achievement. The mother had sent notes to the school giving reasons for some of the absences which included her miscarriage and hospitalization. Some teachers reported that the children showed no interest in school, had excessive dependence on the teacher, or were daydreaming and inattentive. They thought the mother was more interested in her own health than the children's. The 14 and 10-year-old children went to live with an aunt during the mother's hospitalization; the other seven children were cared for at home during the daytime by a homemaker provided by a family agency. There were also many health problems among the children.

From this partial recounting of the needs of the children in this family it is apparent that the energy, scheduling, and time required of the mother to attend to the school and health problems of the children was a burden. In addition limitations in the mother's own health and financial and marital difficulties within the family would cause a strain on any school child. Although this family would appear to have more than its share of problems, it is not unique among the families in the study.

Children in One-Parent Families—Study III

The following is an example of a one-parent family in which three children, ages 6, 9, and 11 years, were doing above average academic work. This family was not dissimilar to the one previously described in the two-parent family. Although marital conflicts in this family were not currently a problem, there had been severe conflicts when the alcoholic father was at home. He had abused and maltreated the children. Although the children were doing above average academic work, the demonstration social worker reported that the children were affected by the mother's mental illness. The school reported that the two older children were somewhat withdrawn, and that the 6-year-old boy was a severe problem in the classroom because he talked out, was impudent, and hit people. The mother visited the school on parents' day in reference to the 6-year-old child but she was unable to talk very much. She felt faint and could not stay to discuss her son's difficulties. Several possibilities for help were discussed with the mother by the demonstration social worker but the mother was unable to follow through although she constantly expressed interest in a plan. The situation steadily deteriorated. In the last two terms of the study year the school work of the oldest child, 11 years old, suffered and her feelings of worthlessness increased. All the children reacted to the turmoil in the home. It was difficult to determine what was accidental and what was deliberate in the injuries to each other and the damage to property both within and outside the home. There was much nagging by the grandmother who reluctantly went to the home to help. This and the inconsistent and inadequate child-care given by the mother created confusion in the children's minds. The mother's threats of placement of the children added to their feelings of insecurity. With such a situation it was surprising that three of the children were reported to be doing above average work in school.

Comparison of Above and Below Academic Standing—Study III

In Study III the number of one-parent and two-parent families was about the same (thirty-two one-parent and thirty-eight two-parent) as was also the number of black families in one-parent (8) and in two-parent families (9). Of the twenty-four children with *above* academic standing, fifteen (62.5%) were of one-parent families while only nine (37.5%) were or two-parent families. Conversely of the thirty-five children with *low* academic standing only nine (26%) were of one-parent families while twenty-six (74%) were of two-parent families. Of the children who had *average* academic standing there was little difference between those of one-parent and those of two-parent families. Thus children of one-parent families had a better over-all academic rating than those of two-parent families, a finding contrary to expectations (Table 7).

Children in one-parent and two-parent families were on the average about the same age except in two instances: (1) the children of one-parent families were on the average a grade above the children of two-parent families; and (2) children of one-parent families in the below average academic standing had a mean age of 8.5 years and a mean grade of 3.4 while children of two-parent families had a mean age of 13.4 years and a mean grade of only 4.2.

Children of sixty-three two-parent and forty-eight one-parent families had repeated grades. Again the children of one-parent families showed up more favorably for 82% were known to have repeated no grades as compared to 51% of the two-parent children. Four of the nine children of one-parent families (44%) who were below average grade had repeated grades while twelve (31%) of the twenty-six children in two-parent families who were below average grade had repeated grades. There were also three children of two-parent families in ungraded classes. Two children of two-parent families in the above average group had repeated a grade.

Fewer children in one-parent families in the above average academic group, as shown in Table 7, had difficulties with child care than children of this group in two-parent families (53% compared with 67%). This was true also in relation to behavioral difficulties in school (47% as compared with 67%). But of the children in the below average academic group, all of the children in one-parent families had difficulties in

TABLE 7
Selected family and personal characteristics of children with above average academic standing by number of parents

| | Academic standing and number of parents | | | | | |
| | Above average | | | Below average | | |
Characteristics	Total children (N = 24)	Two (N = 9)	One (N = 15)	Total children (N = 35)	Two (N = 26)	One (N = 9)
Marital difficulty	25%	67%	0%	54%	73%	0%
Child-care difficulty	58	67	53	91.5	89	100
Supplemental childcare utilized	62	33	80	37	27	67
Behavior difficulties in school	54	67	47	71.5	65	89
Problems of absence or tardiness	33	33	33	34	31	44
Mean age	8.4	8.3	8.4	12.1	13.4	8.5
Mean grade	3.3	2.9	3.6	4	4.2	3.4

child-care and all but one in behavioral problems in school while the number was less in children of two-parent families.

Thus children of one-parent families were more likely to be in the above average academic group and to have somewhat less difficulty both in their child-care problems and in their school behavior than children in two-parent families. When children from one-parent families fell into the below average academic group they tended to have slightly more difficulties than the children of two-parent families.

Behavioral Difficulties in School

Behavioral difficulties as reported by the teachers of these 111 children are shown in Table 8 by number of parents and by interviews at intake to the study and at the end of the study year. The problems are grouped into three categories: (1) neurotic tendencies, (2) agressive or acting-out tendencies, and (3) other category which includes performance-related activities toward school tasks and/or abilities to make friendships among schoolmates. More children both in one-parent and two-parent families were reported to have behavioral difficulties at the end of the year than at the initial interview in the study year. A smaller proportion of children of one-parent families than children in two-parent families had behavioral problems both at the first interview and at the end of the study year. Also there was a slight decrease at the end of the year in the proportion of these problems of children of one-parent families.

The highest incidence of problems was in the grouping of neurotic tendencies (1.2 problems per child). Neurotic tendencies may have been more frequent because of the relatively young average age (8.6 years) of the children. The category of neurotic tendencies had not only the highest number of children but also the highest number of problems per child. Within this category the greatest number of children were withdrawn. In the group showing agressive tendencies, children seeking

TABLE 8
Children with neurotic and aggressive tendencies
and other difficulties as reported by the school
at the initial and year interviews—Study III

| Type of Difficulty | Time of interview and number of parents | | | | | |
| | Initial | | | Year | | |
	Total	Two	One	Total	Two	One
Neurotic tendencies						
Withdrawn	50	35	15	37	26	11
Excessive daydreaming	26	14	12	40	23	17
Inability to concentrate	25	17	8	42	25	17
Excessive dependence on teacher	8	6	2	14	10	4
Total number of problems	109	72	37	133	84	49
Problems per child	1.2	1.3	1.1	1.6	1.6	1.6
Agressive tendencies						
Interrupting class	15	8	7	15	9	6
Attention seeking	20	12	8	25	13	12
Difficulties with peers—bossy	8	6	2	10	4	6
Total number of problems	43	26	17	50	26	24
Problems per child	.5	.5	.5	.6	.6	.6
Other difficulties						
Disinterested in school	23	17	6	23	17	6
Poor study habits	40	27	13	53	35	18
Hard to make friends	16	15	1	17	13	4
Other	7	5	2	24	18	6
Total number of problems	86	64	22	117	83	34
Problems per child	1	1.1	.6	1.4	1.6	1.1
None	21	7	14	29	11	18
Total children with school reports	111	63	48	111	63	48

attention were in the greatest number. In the category of other difficulties, children reported to have poor study habits were the greatest in number. This was true of children of one-parent and two-parent families both at the beginning and end of the study year with one exception: the children of one-parent families at the end of the study year had a larger proportion who showed excessive daydreaming and inability to concentrate than were withdrawn, a difference that may have been due only to the teacher's interpretation of the behavior.

The teachers also reported their evaluation of the emotional adjustment of the 111 children: forty-two (67%) of the sixty-three children of two-parent families were considered well adjusted in contrast to forty-one (85%) of the forty-eight children of one-parent families. Again the children of one-parent families were reported to be doing better, this time in terms of their emotional adjustment. It was surprising, nevertheless, to find the rather high proportion of children who were considered by their teachers to be well adjusted in view of the finding that approximately a third of the children had below average academic standing and approximately three-fourths of the children had at least one behavioral difficulty.

Other difficulties were reported by teachers for twenty-nine (26%) children. They were thought to have physical limitations of sight, hearing, speech, or motor activity which interfered with their normally expected academic achievement. The teachers believed that nearly two-thirds of the children could do better academic work. They also reported that parents were interested or concerned in approximately 45% of the children but expressed marked disinterest in 10% of the schoolchildren. Of the remaining 45% they did not know whether the parents were interested or not. In just over a quarter of the children the school had had no contact with the parents.

Fifty of the total 111 children were known to the demonstration social workers who made some attempts to work with the schools.

However, the social workers gave the following comments about the school service:

School services need to be greatly strengthened. One child sat in school for 7 years without being recognized as needing help. During the year the pupil adjustment counselor in the case was extremely cooperative. However, once planning started for the child to go to a special institution for the mentally retarded, the school wanted immediate placement. This was both unrealistic and impossible. If schools offered the type of services demonstrated as needed by the study, families who denied that problems existed or who refused the help of community services could be faced with the need by an accepted authority, the school. Also, such a social worker in a school with this authority could take action whereas many other agencies have to spend time working through the mother's resistance. If the school had some kind of reaching-out services which began with children in kindergarten and the first grade, many of the children in the study would have been reached many years before and some of the problems prevented.

Certainly one would not dispute the desirability of reaching children before difficulties develop or harden into serious problems. The school provides an opportunity to identify potential problems and to reach children early. These findings suggest that considerably more services to children in the school are required if incipient problems are to be recognized and services provided early.

THE HEALTH OF CHILDREN

In Studies I and II some information concerning the health of children was obtained as a part of the research interviews. Due to difficulties in parents' recall, health conditions may have been underreported. In addition to similar data for Study III, a pediatrician was available to examine the children. The health data, therefore, in Study III is more consistent and complete.

Health of Children in Studies I and II

In Studies I and II private physicians were used more frequently by all families than any other medical resource both before (72.5%) and during the study year (44%). In Study I school health services were most frequently used for the demonstration children (53%); for the control children local health departments (64%) and hospital clinics (27%) were used. Probably these differences were due to the existence of tuberculosis, which has been a traditional concern of health deparments, in the control parents. On the other hand, in Study II a somewhat larger proportion (17%) of demonstration than control (9%) children were seen during the year in hospital clinics. The proportions otherwise were about the same for demonstration and control families in the use of medical resources during the study year.

Children aged 18-21 years in Study I saw a private physician less frequently than those under 18 years in all studies. The same was true for hospital clinics and local health departments. No reason is known for the smaller proportion of children under 18 years in Study II as compared with Study I who were reported to have had contacts with school health services.

No health problems were reported for 64% of the children in Study I and 74% in Study II (Table 9). The most common problems included visual and "other" problems in Study I, frequent colds and speech problems in Study II, and allergies in both studies. The "other" category included a variety of conditions such as congenital hip, thyroid condition, bursitis, chronic constipation, nosebleeds, menstrual difficulties, tonsilitis, "toeing in," flat feet, and one leg shorter than the other. Visual problems and allergies were reported primarily among children aged 6 years and over in both studies. Frequent colds, on the other hand, were most frequently reported for children under 6 years of age, and in Study II for those under 3.

Among the 437 children in the two studies, the largest group (10%) had one or more respiratory infections of an acute type, such as tonsillitis, pneumonia, severe colds, and grippe. Children under the age of 6 were particularly susceptible to these infections. This was also true,

TABLE 9
Children with health problems reported by family
at beginning of the study—Studies I and II

Type of Problem	Age in Years, and Study											
	All		0-2		3-5		6-12		13-17		18-21
	I	II	I	II	I	II	I	II	I	II	I
Vision	18	6	0	1	0	1	5	2	6	2	7
Hearing	3	3	0	1	1	1	2	1	0	0	0
Speech	3	8	1	2	0	4	1	1	1	1	0
Muscular	5	2	0	0	2	1	3	1	0	0	0
Heart	1	3	1	0	0	1	0	0	0	2	0
Bronchial condition	4	2	1	1	0	1	2	0	1	0	0
Over or under weight	2	1	0	0	0	0	1	0	1	1	0
Allergies	14	11	3	0	1	2	6	4	3	5	1
Asthma	6	5	0	1	1	0	5	4	0	0	0
Tuberculosis	3	0	2	0	0	0	1	0	0	0	0
Frequent colds	6	22	2	12	2	4	1	3	1	3	0
Frequent Headaches	1	1	0	0	1	0	0	0	0	1	0
Convulsions	0	5	0	2	0	2	0	1	0	0	0
Taliped (club foot)	2	0	0	0	1	0	0	0	0	0	1
Anemic condition	3	0	1	0	0	0	0	0	1	0	1
Other	12	6	4	1	3	1	2	3	2	1	1
None	124	180	29	40	18	35	44	68	23	37	10
Total children	194	243	41	57	28	47	67	86	39	53	19

as would be expected, of the contagious illnesses of childhood. Seven percent of children among all ages were involved in accidents. Six of the control children, exposed to their parents' tuberculosis, became ill with tuberculosis; five of these were under 6 years of age. Of the 437 children in Studies I and II, 6% were hospitalized because of accidents during the year.

Health of Children in Study III

Children were examined in their homes by a pediatrician on the study staff in fifty-six of the seventy families in Study III. The first examination took place soon after the first research interview at the beginning of the study year and a second examination at the end of the year. Some children were not examined because the parents refused. Among the total of 215 children the pediatrician examined 190 at the first examination and 177 at the end of the year. Most families saw the value of the examination and some expressed their desire for the second examination at the end of the year.

The pediatric examination was designed to obtain information concerning the following: (1) usual sources of health supervision, and medical and dental treatment; (2) height and weight in percentiles; (3) medical history and general health problems of each child; and (4) physical illness of a parent or family history of illnesses. After completion of the examinations the pediatrician gave each mother a written recommendation regarding steps to take for the care of each health problem and for preventive care. At the time of the second examination, the pediatrician evaluated the extent to which the family had carried out his initial recommendations.

Health Supervision

The most frequent source (39%) of health supervision for children less than 6 years of age was the Child Health Clinics of the City. A somewhat larger proportion of one- than two-parent children received their supervision from this source, or from a combination of this source and school services. Even so almost a quarter (22%) of all children under 6 years of age and 17% of those aged 6 years and over had no health supervision; this was a serious neglect of children. About half of the twenty-four black children under 6 years, as compared to one-fifth of the white children, had no health supervision. One-parent black children had the least health supervision. Two-parent black children over 6 years of age had somewhat more health supervision than black children under 6 years because of the school health services which were their only source of health supervision. Similarly, fewer one-parent white children under 6 years had health supervision than two-parent white children under 6 years. In general the proportion of children who received health supervision from a physician was small. A few children of one-parent families and all but one black child had no private physicians.

There was an increase in health supervision during the year of from 12 to 20% of children. More were receiving supervision from hospital clinics at the end of the year. Since all of these changes occurred for both demonstration and control children they are associated with the impact of the initial pediatric examinations and recommendations rather than with the efforts of the demonstration social workers.

Medical Care

In addition to the usual source of health supervision, information was obtained on the usual source of medical care for the children. This was defined as that place from which, or the physician from whom, the child received examination and treatment of illnesses or abnormalities. Only 4% of the children reported to have no source of medical care. Half of all the children and most of the black children received medical care from a public clinic or a combination of sources which included a public clinic. This was probably due to the fact that the services of the public hospital were available without cost to city residents. Only 12% of the families, mostly two-parent families, received their medical care from private physicians exclusively.

Many of the study families had difficulty in carrying out the pediatric recommendations and securing the needed care for the children during the study year. One reason was the need for home help or babysitters to permit the mother to leave the other children to go to the clinic or physician's office. This was especially true for one-parent mothers.

Examination Findings

The height and weight of the children showed no departure from the expected levels for children of their ages.

Basic immunizations had not been completed for 21% of the group of 156 children. Children of one-parent families as well as black children had less adequate immunizations. About half of the one-parent black children had received their immunizations. As would be expected, the largest proportion of children who had not been completely immunized fell in the younger age groups: 68% of the forty-one children 0-2 years as compared to 16% of the fifty-five children aged 3-6 years. Only one of the eighty-one children aged 7 years and over had failed to complete his basic immunizations. This shows the effect of the school health program. Half of the two-parent white children aged 0-2 years and all of the one-parent black children aged 0-2 years failed to complete their immunizations. In the age group 3-5 years more black children than white children had not completed their immunizations, 50% of black children compared with 1.5% of white children.

The most frequent health need found in the pediatric examinations was the need for dental care. Approximately half of the children 3 years and over needed dental care soon and urgently, irrespective of race or number of parents. There was a slight increase in the proportion of adolescent children needing dental care.

Nearly half of the children had had at least one accident and an admission to a hospital, while as many as 28% had had frequent illnesses and 16% more were considered by the pediatrician to be slow in development and learning (Table 10). Frequent illnesses and accidents occurred more often among children under the age of 6, especially for black children, than among older children. Slow development or learning was reported more frequently for children aged 6-17 years than for younger children, perhaps because this condition becomes more evident with age.

Hospitalization had been more frequent at any time in the past among those aged 6-17 years than among the younger children. Of the eighty-seven (49%) children who were hospitalized, twenty-six had a medical problem, eighteen a general surgical one, eight corrective surgery, seven as a result of an accident or injury, and twenty-eight for a combination of these reasons involving one or more admissions.

Major Health Conditions During Year

At the time of the final pediatric examination, information was obtained concerning major illnesses of children during the year, major accidents or injuries, and hospitalizations. A major illness was defined as an illness severe enough to require hospital care or to prevent the child from engaging in his usual activities for more than 48 hours. A similar definition was used for major accidents or injuries. In addition to these major conditions there were many children with other health problems of a minor nature. The distribution of children with a major illness or accident during the year was similar for the various age groups. A total of fourteen children were hospitalized out of 156 in the age group, birth to 12 years. This would correspond to a rate of ninety per 1,000, higher than the rate of the recent National Health Survey

TABLE 10
Five general health problems of children by age and race

Type of Problem	Total children (N = 177)	Age in years, and race			
		0-5		6-17	
		White (N = 63)	Black (N = 17)	White (N = 74)	Black (N = 23)
Frequent illness	28%	33%	47%	26%	9%
Slow development or learning	16	6	12	24	17
Frequent accidents	7	8	18	4	4
Any accident	45	48	53	35	61
Any hospitalization	49	43	23.5	61	48

which reported only fifty hospital discharges per 1,000 in the age group birth to 14 years. Children aged less than 6 were hospitalized more frequently than those 6 years or over.

The type of health problem for which a recommendation was most frequently made by the study pediatrician included those related to vision; skin; bones; joints or muscles; ear, nose and throat; heart; kidneys; bladder; genitalia; nutrition; and "other" problems including allergies, diabetes, malocclusions, behavior difficulties, and mental retardation (Table 11).

Many health problems had been known to the family prior to the pediatric examination but medical care had not been obtained for many of them. Eight children were found to have a possible heart condition of which the family had no prior awareness. Health problems not frequently known to the family included problems of lungs, heart, blood conditions, and hernias.

Some action was taken by parents in the majority of instances in which a recommendation was made. In every instance when recommendations to continue or resume treatment were made action was taken. When recommendations to investigate a problem that had not previously been under treatment were made the response of families

TABLE 11
Number of children with health problems and pediatric recommendations

Type of Problem	No recommendation	Total with recommendations	Continue or resume treatment	Investigate possible problem	
				Known to family	Unknown to family
Vision	159	18	9	7	2
Hearing	170	7	5	2	0
Speech	172	5	1	4	0
Skin	166	11	7	2	2
Bones, joints, muscles	167	10	4	5	1
Eyes	173	4	2	2	0
Ears, nose, throat	162	15	5	8	2
Lungs	171	6	2	1	3
Heart	168	9	1	0	8
Stomach, intestine	175	2	2	0	0
Kidneys, bladder, genitalia	159	18	4	10	4
Blood	171	6	1	2	3
Hernia	170	7	0	3	4
Nutrition	162	15	0	12	3
Other	137	40	11 (a)	23 (b)	6
Total children	177	177	177	177	177

(a) Includes one child who also had a recommendation to investigate a possible problem known to family.

(b) Includes two children who also had a recommendation to investigate a possible problem unknown to family.

was not uniform. Action for treatment of problems of vision, skin, kidneys, bladder, genitalia, and hernia was not usually taken.

At the time of examination the pediatrician made an over-all health rating of each child. A child with serious or multiple health problems was rated as poor; one with some health problems as fair; and one with minor or no health problems as good. Of the 177 children examined 83% had a rating of fair, 11% of good, and 6% of poor. Of interest is the fact that a higher percentage of children of one-parent families, particularly black children, had a rating of good. Conversely a higher percentage of two-parent black children had ratings of poor than two-parent white children. There were no differences among the several age groups except for those aged 13-17 years who had more ratings of good than poor or fair. None of these differences, however, were statistically significant.

Between the first and second pediatric examination 8.5% of the 177 children improved in their health ratings and 5% had deteriorated. The latter group was evenly distributed between demonstration and control children which suggests that no over-all improvement in the health status of children was brought about by the demonstration social workers.

At the time of the yearly examination, the pediatrician rated the performance of the family in regard to the action taken during the year on the recommendations made at the first examination (Table 12). The rating was done on a three point scale. Families were assessed as (1) having adequately handled or followed through the initial recommendation to secure further examination or treatment, (2) having made some but not sufficient effort to follow through or having followed through on some but not all, or (3) having failed to follow through on recommendations.

The response to the pediatric recommendations was widespread. The family failed to take action in regard to 26% of the children. This was true, however, of 52% of the twenty-five two-parent black children as

TABLE 12
Family health performance rating for demonstration and control children

Follow-up on pediatric recommendations	Total Children	Number of parents and race			
		Two		One	
		White	Black	White	Black
All children	(N = 177)	(N = 76)	(N = 25)	(N = 61)	(N = 15)
Adequate	30%	34%	16%	30%	33%
Partial	37	44	20	39	27
None	26	18	52	26	20
Other (a)	7	4	12	5	20
Demonstration children	(N = 82)	(N = 34)	(N = 10)	(N = 32)	(N = 6)
Adequate	28%	25.5%	10%	28%	83%
Partial	44	53	10	50	17
None	22	17.5	50	22	0
Other (a)	6	6	30	0	0
Control children	(N = 95)	(N = 42)	(N = 15)	(N = 29)	(N = 9)
Adequate	32%	43%	20%	31%	0%
Partial	32	36	27	28	33
None	29	19	53	31	33
Other (a)	7	2	0	10	33

(a) Unable to rate, unknown, or no health problems.

compared to only 18% of the seventy-six two-parent white children ($X^2 = 9.1$, p $<$ .01). Both the demonstration and the control children contributed about equally to this difference.

Some differences between demonstrations and controls do appear, however, among the one-parent black children. The recommendations were adequately followed up in five out of six (83%) one-parent black children in the demonstration as compared with none of the nine controls in black families. This difference suggests that the services of the demonstration improved the health status of these children. On the other hand, a somewhat larger proportion of two-parent white control families than of the two-parent demonstration families followed recommendations adequately, but the difference is not large enough to be significant. When families did not follow through, the most frequent reason given by the families was that they did not consider them important. Other reasons given were the cost of care and the time involved.

In order to examine whether sibling size and children's ages were associated with the family health performance rating, the 177 children were first divided into a group of fifty-six children living in families in which there were less than four children and a second group of 121 children in families of four or more children. Those families with less than four children adequately followed up the recommendations more frequently than families with four or more children: 45% of the children in families with less than four children as compared with 23% in families of four children or more ($X^2 = 7.4$, p $<$ .01).

SUMMARY

Children were involved in the disturbances caused by the mental illness of parents more than they were by those associated with the tuberculous condition of parents. This was accounted for by a period of time allowed the tuberculous parents to prepare for hospitalization and by the differences in the behavior of parents with these two illnesses Over half of the children in each study were involved in the illnesses but a quarter more in the urban study: 80% of the children of mothers who went to the emergency services were affected by their mothers' mental illness. Even in the families which reported no involvement of children the research data indicated this was not necessarily so. These were most often children in the preschool years.

The difficulties of the children were divided into behavioral difficulties and neurotic traits. Over half of the children (52%) were reported to have no difficulties. Again children of mentally ill parents had more of these difficulties than children of tuberculous parents. Otherwise the proportions of difficulties for children in the three studies were strikingly similar. More families reported neurotic type difficulties than behavioral difficulties. There was no significant difference in the three studies between one-parent or two-parent families.

A lower proportion of children of one-parent families had repeated grades than those of two-parent families. More black children had repeated grades than white children. It was surprising to find from the school reports that the proportion of children with above grade placement tended to be higher for children of one-parent families than for children of two-parent families. Also a higher proportion were at grade placement and a lower proportion at below grade placement than in two-parent families. These differences may be related to severe marital discord frequently reported in two-parent families.

In the children with above average academic standing there were other interesting and unexpected differences between children of one- and two-parent families. Although the average age of the children was the same, children of one-parent families were somewhat further advanced in grade level than the children of two-parent families. Children of one-parent families also had fewer repeated grades and fewer of them were reported by their teachers to be not well adjusted. Also fewer of the one-parent children were reported by the teachers to have difficulties in their home situations, including child-care problems, than children in two-parent families.

Efforts of the demonstration social workers were primarily focused on problems in the home and the care of children and secondarily on the children's school difficulties. The need for early school identification and help to families with problems affecting children was clear.

In the surburban studies, one-half to three-quarters of children were reported to have no health problem. These families used private physicians for the medical care of their children while in the urban study half of all the children and most of the black children received medical care in public clinics. In the urban study a pediatrician on the study staff examined most of the children. These children had most of their health care in city health clinics and school health services. A quarter of all the children and half of the black children under 6 years had had no health supervision. The physical examination showed height and weight of the children were at the expected levels for children of their ages. Almost a quarter of the children had not completed their immunizations and this was higher for preschool children. The most frequent and urgent health need was for dental care. There was a large variety of other health problems including accidents and malnutrition known and unknown to parents. Only 11% of the children were rated as having good health. There were differences in the number of families who followed through on the pediatricians' recommendations according to parent status, number of children, and race, but only a quarter of all parents failed to take some action on the pediatric recommendations.

6

Provisions for Care

With the mental hospitalization of a parent, especially a mother, the family was forced to make plans for the supervision and care of the children. Children in these families of hospitalized parents had the same types of risks as other children whose fathers or mothers were absent from the home because of separation, divorce, death, or other reasons. However, in addition, these children had the added risks of having a parent who was ill for a shorter or longer period of time before the hospital admission. Usually the family had no clear indication, nor could one usually be given at the time of admission, of the duration of the parent's hospital stay; thus, this uncertainty made planning for satisfactory child care more difficult for the family.

Data from the pilot Study I showed that the most obvious disruption in the living arrangements of children of hospitalized parents involved separations of the children from their usual environment. Separation from their own homes, therefore, as well as separation from their ill parents, frequently occurred when the parents were hospitalized. This separation often involved, also, separations from their other parent, separations from their siblings, school peers, or their own neighborhood or community. The impact of the separation from home was often, therefore, a major separation from all that was familiar. It often created an uncertainty for the child as to the reason for the separation and the length of it.

Another finding from Study I showed that disruptions in the living arrangements of children were common in families with parental hospitalization for physical illness (tuberculosis) and mental illness. There were three factors that consistently determined the extent of the disruption: (1) the hospitalization of the mother caused considerably more disruption in the living arrangements and care of the children than the hospitalization of the father; (2) the children of one-parent families experienced the greatest disruption and, since these were also families of a hospitalized mother, the children were left without a parent upon her hospital admission; and (3) families varied greatly from those with adequate supplemental or substitute resources to those with few or no resources.

In Study I although the number of families in the tuberculosis group was small, the proportions of families with separations of children were essentially the same as in the mental illness group in both the one- and two-parent families. The separation of children in both families with mental illness and tuberculosis was largely dependent upon such factors as the parental composition of the family, ages of children, availability of relatives, or other resources. However, there were other factors that differentiated the two hospital groups that tended to make it somewhat less distressful for the families in the control (tuberculosis) group to plan for the care of their children. Briefly stated, these differentiating factors included:

1) In the case of admission of a parent to a tuberculosis sanatorium, there was usually a period of at least 2 to 3 weeks prior to the scheduled admission date when the ill parent and family, together, could make at least preliminary arrangements for the maintenance of the family, including the care of the children during the parent's hospitalization. In contrast, the admission of a parent to a mental hospital was frequently prompted by critical, disruptive, or deviant behavior, resulting in an apparently abrupt and sudden decision for hospitalization.

2) In the case of admission of a parent to a tuberculosis sanatorium,

the patients accepted hospitalization more readily, though not, of course, without reluctance, in terms of protection for their families and in the belief that they were doing something which ultimately favored the family health and solidarity. On the other hand, the admission of a parent to a mental hospital was accompanied often by the strong resistance of the patient to accept hospitalization, sometimes to the point of involving the local police or court. This made an already difficult situation worse and interfered with planning for the care of the children.

3) In the case of admission of a parent to a tuberculosis sanatorium, the patient and family were usually told the expected length of hospitalization. In contrast, upon admission to a mental hospital, the patient and family were seldom able to plan on the length of hospitalization, which again complicated their planning for family maintenance and care of the children.

4) In the case of a parent's hospitalization for tuberculosis, the duration of the hospitalization was almost twice as long as in families with mental hospitalization. Over one-half of the tuberculous patients had 6 months or more of hospitalization, whereas, 80% of mentally ill patients were discharged within 3 months, and 20% of those were readmitted within the next 3 months. In addition, when the mentally ill patient returned to his home the family often accepted him with hesitancy and increased anxiety since many symptoms of the illness were still present, while the families of tuberculous patients had confidence that the parent was well again.

Separation

The studies focused on the separations of children from their homes because of the hospitalization of a parent, but included also a substantial number of separations from home for reasons other than parental hospitalizations. In spite of differences in the three studies, the proportions of families with at least one child separated from home during the study period were similar. Children were separated in approximately one-third of the two-parent families and two-thirds of the one-parent families.

1) Study I initially examined the plans made for the care and living arrangements of the children 6 weeks after the parent's hospitalization. The control group was comprised of parents hospitalized for tuberculosis and the demonstration group, of parents hospitalized for mental illness.

2) Study II initially examined the plans for the children as soon as possible after the parent's mental hospitalization with the hope of lessening the extent of separation of children in the demonstration group through the intervention and coordination of existing community and hospital services. The control families received no interventive service from the study. The control group was largely suburban families as opposed to families in two small cities in the demonstration group.

3) Study III initially examined the plans for children as soon as possible after the mother's visit to the psychiatric emergency services. Only thirty-four (49%) of the seventy mothers in this study were hospitalized during the study year (largely for psychiatric reasons). Most of the demonstration and control families were living in a large city and were of low socioeconomic status. The demonstration by the study staff aimed primarily to lessen the proportion of children separated from their homes. The control group received no help from the study staff except the recommendations of the pediatrician who examined the children.

In spite of the different emphases in the three studies, the proportions of families with children separated from their homes for any reason were the same. When fathers were hospitalized there were no separations of children from their homes in any of the three studies, since mothers were able to keep the home intact and the children with them. For these reasons, the further data describes separation of children with ill mothers rather than with ill fathers.

In the total of 199 families with ill mothers about one-half of the families had children who were separated from their own homes (eighty-seven or 44%). One-parent families with ill mothers had a higher proportion of children separated (64%) than the two-parent families (32%). This difference was maintained in all three studies. The proportion of children separated from their homes was lowest in the urban study (Study III) than in the studies in small cities and suburban areas (Studies I and II). Even though there were more one-parent families in Study III than in the other two studies, the difference between the studies was probably due to the fact that only half of the mothers in Study III were hospitalized during the study year whereas a parent was hospitalized in each family in Studies I and II and more often this was the mother.

There was a marked similarity in Studies I and II in the proportions of families with at least one child separated from home. Families living in small cities and suburban areas made greater use of homes of relatives and friends for the care of children than did families in the urban areas; yet, the problems in urban families were frequently more severe than those in the suburban families. Of the total of 199 ill mothers, 44% had children separated from home. Of these 22% were separated primarily because of the mother's hospitalization and 20% for reasons other than the mother's hospitalization. About the same number of children in demonstration families as in control families were separated. However in all three studies about twice as many more one-parent families than two-parent families had children separated. As would be expected because of the hospitalization of mothers in Studies I and II, those studies had more families with children separated than Study III when most mothers were not hospitalized (Table 13).

Forty-three (26%) of the 163 mothers who were hospitalized had

TABLE 13
Families of ill mothers with separation of children from home:
a. For any reason
b. For reasons other than hospitalization of mother

	Study and number of parents in family								
	Total families			I		II		III	
	Both	Two	One	Two	One	Two	One	Two	One
Total study	(N = 190)	(N = 125)	(N = 74)	(N = 34)	(N = 20)	(N = 53)	(N = 22)	(N = 38)	(N = 32)
a. Any reason	44%	32%	64%	35%	70%	38%	68%	21%	56%
b. Other than mother's hospitalization	20	14	28	6	20	17	18	18	41
Demonstration	(N = 103)	(N = 58)	(N = 45)	(N = 24)	(N = 14)	(N = 15)	(N = 15)	(N = 19)	(N = 6)
a. Any reason	44%	28%	65%	37%	71%	33%	60%	11%	63%
b. Other than mother's hospitalization	17	9	29	8	29	13	7	5	50
Control	(N = 96)	(N = 67)	(N = 29)	(N = 10)	(N = 6)	(N = 38)	(N = 7)	(N = 19)	(N = 16)
a. Any reason	44%	36%	62%	30%	67%	40%	86%	32%	50%
b. Other than mother's hospitalization	22	19	28	0	0	18	43	32	31

repeated hospitalizations for mental or physical illnesses during the time of the studies (6 months in Study I, and a year in Studies II and III). These forty-three mothers had 104 hospitalizations ranging from two to five hospitalizations for each mother. In all these hospitalizations of ill mothers the families had to plan for the care of the children.

In Study I, the families used homemaker services only when the families themselves sought those services. In Study II homemakers were offered to the demonstration group through the demonstration community committee but only after the hospitalization of the mother had occurred. The families had often made other child-care plans before the demonstration social worker saw the family. Frequently the families left the children with relatives just prior to taking the patient to the hospital or even on their way to the hospital. For subsequent hospitalizations, the families often preferred to utilize relatives for child-care even when homemaker services were offered. In Study III of the nineteen two-parent families eleven of these mothers were hospitalized, and the demonstration worker was able to secure homemaker services in five of these, thereby avoiding separation of the children. In the sixteen one-parent families with mothers hospitalized, only one family had a homemaker provided. This showed the limited use of homemakers in one-parent families and the difficulty of keeping children at home when the only parent, the mother, was hospitalized.

In the T family, the demonstration social worker prevented separation of children from the home during a second hospitalization of a mother in a two-parent family. Mrs. T. was a 27-year-old mother of two children, ages 5 and 2 years, who was hospitalized in the psychiatric ward of a general hospital a few days after her initial visit to the emergency service where she received a diagnosis of psychotic depressive reaction. She complained of not being able to cope with the care of her children. She felt housework was too much for her, stating:

For the last few weeks, I have felt weak and I have neglected my children. After my operation [4 months previously for aneurysm] we moved to a new apartment and nothing has gone right. The toilet broke, the kitchen sink leaks, the back door is broken, and everything has gone wrong. I have no patience at all with my children and scream at them all the time. I am worried that my girl, the 5-year-old, knows something is wrong with me. I know I frighten the children by screaming. I am different from what I was before my operation.

Her husband was worried about her statements that she could no longer be a good wife and that there was no point to her living. She also had made a suicidal gesture by taking several unknown pills. She complained of headaches, loss of sleep, feeling tired all the time, weakness, and was very apathetic and discouraged.

Six months prior to the Study, this mother had been hospitalized for surgery. Her brother and his wife then took the two children to live with them. During the hospitalization for mental illness, he took the 2-year-old and the husband's sister took the 5-year-old. The two children were separated from one another because her brother did not want to take both children for the third time. Although Mrs. T. had four married sisters living in the vicinity, she had had no contact with them and would not ask them to help with the children's care. Actually, her mother and one unmarried sister lived in the downstairs apartment, but their relationship was not always good (her mother had a long history of alcoholism) so there was little possibility of their help.

After 7½ weeks of hospitalization in the psychiatric ward of the general hospital, Mrs. T. was transferred to a state hospital. After a few days in the state hospital, she left against medical advice "because I couldn't stand the place." The demonstration social worker visited Mrs. T. weekly after she left the state hospital. Mrs. T. accepted very well the emotional support given by the demonstration social worker in relation to child-care and housekeeping responsibilities, but was threatened whenever problems of a more substantive nature were discussed. Shortly after her return home, she had become pregnant although she stated she did not want another child at this time. She was, therefore, hospitalized later in the year for the birth of her third child. At this time, the demonstration social worker obtained a homemaker and the two children remained at home.

Although this case presents the situation of a family with many relatives available for substitute child care, there were definite limitations in their time or willingness to accept the added responsibility and expense required to care for other than their own children. Only a few families offered or were able to pay their own relatives for the expense involved in caring for their children even when a relative gave up a job to serve as a substitute caretaker.

The N. family in contrast to the T. family had for a long time been burdened with severe marital conflict. Mrs. N. was a 40-year-old mother of six children aged 19 to 6 years. Only four of the children were at home because the two oldest girls had left home, one to be married and the other to work in California. Mrs. N.'s mental illness and the father's severe alcoholism resulted in frequent abusiveness to his wife and children.

Mrs. N. had four hospitalizations during the study year, three for mental illness and the other for the delivery of her seventh child, an unwanted pregnancy. At her emergency visit, Mrs. N. complained that her husband had beaten her for 20 years and kept her hostage. She showed bruises on her arms and stated he abused her and the children, especially when he was intoxicated. She stated that she read the Bible all the time and that recently she had heard her dead father's voice. The diagnosis given at her emergency visit was acute schizophrenia, paranoid type. She was sent home from the emergency service with her husband and advised to go to the state hospital the following day. She was hospitalized for about 2 weeks. At this time, she was given a diagnosis of personality trait disturbance—passive aggressive personality, passive dependent type—with marked anxiety, delusions about communication with God, and hallucinations.

The youngest child, a 6-year-old boy, was sent to live with a cousin. Mrs. N. was dissatisfied with these arrangements during her hospitalization. During her second hospitalization of about 1 week, and her third hospitalization for the birth of her child, a neighbor offered to care for the 6-year-old boy. The newborn child at 1 month of age was seen by the visiting nurse because of vomiting. The nurse thought the mother was nervous and held the baby too tightly during feedings. She was concerned about the mother's mental health and the father's excessive drinking. The mother resisted efforts of the visiting nurse and the demonstration social worker to help her.

Mrs. N.'s fourth mental hospitalization was caused by her bizarre behavior when she suddenly ingested a number of orinase pills (belonging to her diabetic mother-in-law who was visiting), slashed her wrists, and started a fire in the house all within the same day. She was hospitalized for 6 weeks and during this time was comatose for several days. A short time prior to this episode, the 19-year-old married daughter was called home from California to help with the children.

She had obtained a job in the vicinity, but was very reluctant to stay out of work for a few days until the demonstration social worker could arrange homemaker services because she needed the money. A homemaker was accepted by the family. This gave an opportunity for better understanding of the many destructive factors constantly present in this family. With a homemaker present, the 6-year-old child remained in his own home.

The following family illustrates how older children separate themselves from the turmoil and conflict within a home.

In the Y. family, the two older daughters left the home as soon as they could get out. The 17-year-old boy went off for days or weeks at a time to live with friends because he felt home conditions were intolerable. The demonstration social worker reported him to be an angry, bitter young man who tended to isolate himself from the family. In a discussion with the demonstration social worker, he blamed his father for all the problems in the family and stated with much hostility that because he, the boy, had had a difficult life he planned to make it difficult for everyone else. It was impossible to engage him in any thoughtful planning for his future, although at times he had expressed a desire to go to college to study engineering. At the time of the study, he was involved in an engineering apprentice course in a local shipbuilding company.

The demonstration social worker reported that there were severe marital conflicts in this family related largely to the father's alcoholism and the rather shattered parent-child relationships over a length of time. Little or no improvement in this family situation was seen nor could any have been expected by the end of 1 year. The introduction of the homemaker was one of the most effective aids offered the family, although a great deal of effort was put into the family by medical and social agencies.

Separation of Children for Reasons Other Than Mother's Illness

In addition to children who were separated from their families because of the hospitalization of their mothers, in an unexpectedly high proportion of families (20%), children were separated for reasons other than hospitalization. The proportion of families that had at least one child separated during the study year increased from Study I (11%) to Study III (29%). The proportion of two-parent families in which children were separated for other reasons was similar in all three studies but the proportions were consistently lower in the two-parent families (14%) as opposed to 28% in the one-parent families. The children of one-parent families, therefore, had experienced more separations from their homes whether because of the hospitalization of the mother or for other reasons.

Of the thirty-eight demonstration families with mothers hospitalized with mental illness in Study I, there were six families where children were separated for reasons other than the mother's illness. In the sixteen families with mothers hospitalized with tuberculosis there were no instances of children separated for other reasons.

In Study III there was an interesting and significant difference between the one- and two-parent demonstration families; only one (5%) of the two-parent families had a child separated for other reasons as opposed to eight (50%) of the one-parent families. The difference may be accounted for by the demonstration itself since there were four of these eight one-parent families in which the demonstration social worker encouraged the family to place the children with children's agencies while in one family the worker actually instigated the separation.

In this case Mrs. P. was a white, 22-year-old, twice divorced mother of a 1-year-old child with a severe disturbance in the mother-child relationship. The demonstration social worker instigated, early in the study year, the placement of the child through the public child welfare department because of suspected neglect and abuse of the child. The mother readily admitted that she had never wanted this child and often felt hostile toward her, expressing fear at the time of her emergency visit that she was going to harm the child. The child had a history of many falls, had been hospitalized several times for question of fractures and seizures, and also had by accident swallowed some room deodorizer. Early in the study year, the child was admitted for dehydration and seizures. During the period of the mother's own hospitalization for a personality disorder, the child was cared for by the maternal grandparents. The mother and her child often lived in the maternal grandparents' home. The mother stated several times: "My baby gets on my nerves—sometimes I feel like throwing her out of the window—and sometimes I feel like jumping too!" The child was placed in a foster home following the child's hospitalization for a fall and seizures. In spite of many efforts on the mother's part to avoid the placement plan, the demonstration social worker, the child welfare agency, and other social and health agencies were able to convince her of the child's need for continued placement.

A substantial proportion of mothers reported difficulties in their relationships with their children or in their ability to cope with their care. Separations for these reasons involved a variety of situations ranging from serious problems requiring long-term institutional care or foster-home placement to situations of lesser severity and duration. Whereas the separation of children from their homes when related to the hospitalization of the mother resulted from a lack or absence of any adequate supplemental child-care resources *within* the home, such as a relative or homemaker, the separations of children from their homes for reasons other than the mother's hospitalization were, for the most part, related to the inability of the mother to provide adequate care for her children *when* she was at home. Severe disturbances in parent-child relationships and in the distress associated with parental mental illness were often the reasons why care of children elsewhere was necessary. Usually an older child in the family left the home temporarily or permanently to avoid a distressful parental relationship.

An example of severe mother-child relationships resulting in separation of children from home is the C. family, a control case. Mrs. C., a 42-year-old mother with three daughters, aged 19, 18, and 15 years, on her fourth visit to the psychiatric emergency service within 1½ years was given a diagnosis of adult situational reaction. She was described as returning to the emergency service with the same problem as before and had refused to keep psychiatric outpatient appointments. She stated her home situation was bad and she had to get out of it. She reported that 2 days before her visit, her two older daughters had left the house because "We had a big fight." In the initial research interview, Mrs. C. stated that she and her husband "fight all the

time—every day—and I know that's the reason my girls left the house.
They have gone to live with my sister-in-law. They are both going to be
married in a few weeks, and I know it is partly because they can't stand
me. They have known something is wrong with me. I cry all the time,
and I have tried to commit suicide six times in the past year" (one
attempt with barbiturates, a serious attempt by slashing her wrists with
mirror glass, another attempt with a knife, and once by throwing
herself down the stairs).

By the time of the four-month research interview, this mother had
again attempted suicide which resulted in a 2-week period in a hospital.
During this time, her 15-year-old daughter was alone during the day
until her father returned from work. This child had been showing severe
school problems, and on the day of her sixteenth birthday dropped out
of school. Shortly thereafter, she separated herself from the family and
soon was married to get out of the house for good.

This type of separating from the family when the child preferred to
live elsewhere occurred more often with the older children. Some of the
separations were serious with intentions never to return. Others were
less serious, often of short duration, and occurred more frequently.
Some children who returned to their own homes after living with
relatives during their mother's hospitalization preferred to live with
their relatives, especially when the mother's behavior was still upsetting
to them.

Another reason for separation was the mother's inability to cope with
the care of her children. These were usually younger children whose
development depended on the mother's ability to give good care.

A striking example of this was the control case of Mrs. S., a
25-year-old mother of four children, aged 6, 3, 1 year, and 4 months.
During Mrs. S.'s 2-week hospitalization for anemia (and hysterical
features), her mother-in-law cared for the children until their father
returned from work. This was unsatisfactory because of the mother-in-
law's alcoholism. Attempts were made to find other care for these
children but they were unsuccessful. As a result Mrs. S. left the hospital
against medical advice. Soon after she returned home, she found that
she could not cope with the children's care. She relied heavily on the
6-year-old child to help with the care of the younger children. This
child had been trained also to use the phone, to dial Operator, and to

ask the police to transfer her mother to the hospital whenever the mother felt ill and was fearful of having a blackout. The research interviewer reported that the mother had visited the emergency service frequently, especially during the previous 2 years. Although Mrs. S. was hospitalized only once during the study year, she reported increasing difficulties in taking care of her children. In addition the children were having serious medical problems and the husband had surgery. Mr. S. finally drove the children to his parents in North Carolina because no one else was able to take care of them. The children stayed with their grandparents for 2 months when Mr. S. brought them home. Separation, therefore, was due not because of the hospitalization of the mother, but because of the mother's inability to cope with their care.

Age of Children

Children in the age group 0-2 years were separated from their homes more frequently than children older than 2 years both in one-parent and two-parent families. In the preschool ages 0-5 years of age over half of the children were separated; this was somewhat higher in two-parent families with mothers ill (67%) than in one-parent families with mothers ill (56%). In the school aged years (6-17 years) almost twice as many children were separated in one-parent families (52%) as in two-parent families (26%). The problems associated with separation were therefore greater for the infants and preschool children. Among the older children separations were more permanent than temporary.

Since children in the age group 6 through 17 years were school children, their families often hoped that plans could be made so that the children could remain in their own homes and thereby not have to change schools. Families often viewed the separation of the child from his school as a more serious separation than from his own home. The preschool age groups of 0-2 and 3-5 years, however, did not have this reason for keeping the child in his own home. The problem of these age periods was the need of the young child for total care. Unless there was someone available to give daytime care in the home until the father could take over the responsibilities after his working hours, the preschool child was usually separated from his home and cared for elsewhere during the mother's hospitalization. Thus, the younger children were more frequently separated from their homes than older children.

Changes in Child Care

Frequently the children could not stay with relatives throughout the mothers' hospitalizations (Table 14). Several changes in child-care took place. There was an interesting difference between those families in which children were not separated from their homes and those families in which children were separated from their homes when mothers were hospitalized. When children were separated combinations of plans or multiple child-care arrangements were carried out in twenty-four (35%) of the families. These twenty-four families were about equally divided between one-parent families and two-parent families, and between demonstration and control families. Eight of these twenty-four mothers were readmitted within the study year. The child-care arrangements in subsequent hospitalizations did not improve except in three demonstration families in Study III which used homemakers.

In ten families foster homes or institutional care was used for the children because of the mother's hospitalization. Seven of these ten families were control families and half of the ten were one-parent families.

Child care by relatives was often questionable or uncertain because of the length of the mother's hospitalization or, in some families, because the patient's children and the relative's children did not get along together. This involved sending the children to another relative's home or siblings were shifted to different homes. In at least 61% of the families with children placed, siblings were divided among relatives. Some families recognized that repeated changes created difficult

TABLE 14
Caretaking situations for children in 163 families of hospitalized mothers

	No separation		Separation	
	Families with no children separated (all children cared for in own home)		Families with children separated (at least one child cared for in other than own home)	
Relatives regularly living in home	21	(22%)	Children in relatives' homes — 37	(55%)
Relatives to home for temporary child-care	12	(13%)	Children to homes of neighbors or friends — 3	(4%)
Father at home (unemployed or stayed home from work)	8	(8%)	Children placed in foster homes — 3	(4%)
Father home after work	44	(46%)	Combinations and multiple child-care arrangements — 24	(35%)
Children alone after school	(19)	(20%)	Total families — 68	(100%)
Part-time substitute care	(15)	(16%)		
Daytime paid help (i.e., baby-sitter, housekeeper)	(6)	(6%)		
Homemaker	(4)	(4%)		
Combinations and multiple child-care arrangements	10	(11%)		
Total families	95	(100%)		

adjustments for the child, while others felt that all the children needed were bed and board.

For example, the W. family expressed a need only for financial assistance; yet, the family had many other problems including an unusual variety of child-care plans. Mrs. W., a 33-year-old, twice married woman (divorced and remarried to the same man), was the mother of three children, 9-year-old twin girls and a 4-year-old girl. The father in this family was in a correctional institution because of alcoholism and had been in jails and hospitals many times. He had not worked for the previous ten years. During most of the time, the family had been supported by Public Assistance. On Christmas Day, the patient's father-in-law visited the home because he had learned the children had no Christmas gifts. He broke down the door because he smelled gas and found the patient with her head in the oven and her left wrist slashed. The children were in bed, were hysterical, and said that their mother had been telling strange stories and imagining people were lurking around her. The patient later admitted that she had been carrying a knife for protection for over 3 weeks.

The patient was taken by Police to the local General Hospital from which she was transferred to a mental hospital. The father-in-law bundled up the three children and distributed them among the relatives; he reluctantly took the twins and the 4-year-old was kept by the aunt. After 2 weeks, there was a complete shift in living arrangements. The grandparents said that they "had had it" and "felt that the aunt should take all three children." She again refused to do this because of her own three children; so the twins went to another aunt who had five children. The aunt stated: "My conscience began to bother me, so I took one twin for a while; the other one stayed where she was, and the 4-year-old who had been with me went to another aunt because she and my son fought constantly. I feel that the twin that is with me now needs attention because she refuses to eat, has frequent nausea, cries a lot, and won't go to bed alone. I am concerned, also, that her wild fears will rub off onto my children. I feel sorry for the children, but I have just about had enough myself; yet, we just couldn't put them into state homes." In a later interview with the mother, she felt that it was probably "a little hard on the children to move to a new environment, but they would adjust easily to these things. We have been receiving Public Assistance to maintain our apartment while I was in the hospital, so everything has worked out just fine." The mother at this time had returned home after 3 months in a hospital; her husband had also returned home and the three children were back with them.

The mother in this family obviously minimized the disruptive experiences for her children during her hospitalization. Her psychiatrist recommended that one 9-year-old twin be seen by a child guidance clinic. The relatives, on the other hand, although recognizing that these changes in child-care plans were difficult for the children, felt that their own situations and responsibilities necessitated them. Each of the three children in the family was separated from each other at one time or another as well as changing homes. The twins in the third grade in school had both repeated the first grade and were transferred to two or three different schools within 6 months.

In families in which some children remained in the same home of a relative throughout the mother's hospitalization, there were, also, some complications involved.

The relatives of Mrs. X. never accepted the mother's mental illness, believing it was just an excuse for the mother to shirk her responsibility of caring for the children. Mrs. X., a 22-year-old mother with three children, aged 3, 2 years, and 10 months, was hospitalized for the third time 4 weeks after the birth of the youngest child. She had had depressive symptoms just before the birth of this child and 6 days following delivery stated that she wanted to die. Prior to her mental hospitalization, she stayed in bed most of the time, did not want to care for her children, and neglected their care. Upon her admission, her husband's parents took the two oldest children and her sister-in-law, who had three small children of her own, took the infant. The 22-year-old father lived with his parents and his children during the 8-week hospitalization to "try to help with the children's care; my mother wasn't too well and she couldn't do it all alone." He also tried to help whenever he was able with the care of the infant because "my sister-in-law started to get a little nasty about having the baby. She felt my wife could take care of the children if she really wanted to." Between this young father's efforts to ease his relatives' care of his three children and his frequent visits to the hospital, he stated, "I began to get things mixed up on my job." The grumblings of both his mother and sister-in-law about caring for his children finally prompted him to request foster-home placement from the welfare department. In the meantime, his wife heard of his plan and said, "Although I didn't feel ready to leave the hospital, I went home to prevent my children from being boarded out. It upset me terribly to know our relatives had to take care of the children. It upset me even more to think of their going to a foster home, so I left the hospital." After 3 months at home, this mother was readmitted to the mental hospital, again complaining of not being able to care for her children and again being very upset because her relatives were involved in the children's care.

Relatives of some families were faced with serious situations when they took the children into their own homes. Sometimes this meant rearrangement of their living quarters, particularly bedrooms. In two families, they planned to build on one other additional bedroom because their quarters were too small. These relatives felt the children should not return home when the mothers came out of the hospital. Some mothers moved in with relatives after discharge from the hospital.

It was not uncommon that the relatives' willingness to help out with the children was related to the understanding which they had of the mother's mental illness and with their past experiences in caring for the children. They sometimes were frightened by it, feared it, avoided it, or were sympathetic to it, and sometimes "fed up" with it, or they even denied it. Such reactions did not usually affect a relative's readiness to take over the care of the patient's children but they probably did affect the care in some instances. Relatives played, however, a major role in the substitute care of the children, not only in the relatives' homes but in the children's own home. Among the ninety-five families with no separation of children, as many as 22% of the families had relatives living regularly in their homes. These relatives, for the most part, were the grandmothers of the children and were acquainted with their care and the routines of the home. This minimized the disruption. Many relatives had frequently filled in for substitute care. There were 13% of the families in which a relative, usually the grandmother, was available and willing to move into the home for the duration of the hospitalization. Therefore relatives in over one-third of the families with ill mothers were either in the home or moved into the home to care for the children and thereby prevent the need for their separation.

Child-care in these instances provided consistent care throughout the duration of the hospitalization. When a fifth of these mothers were readmitted during the study year the relatives provided the same substitute child-care as before.

Grandmothers had frequently helped their daughters prior to hospitalization and were particularly likely to do this following childbirth or during other periods of stress. Among the families of relatively young mothers, grandmothers were a major resource for child-care. In families of older patients, an older child assisted in the household duties or in the care of younger siblings when the mother was incapacitated.

The presence of older children in the home also influenced the nature of the child-care role of the father during the mother's hospitalization. In eight families the fathers stayed home to care for their children. These eight families had 2.5 children each, all except two of whom were under 12 years of age. In most of these families with children (19) over 12 years of age, the fathers cared for the children after work. These children were old enough to care for themselves for short periods of time and also to assume some responsibility for younger siblings. In six families, the older children stayed out of school on occasion to care for the younger children in the family whenever a housekeeper or relative could not come because of illness or other emergencies.

A particularly blatant example of this is the D. family, a control case. Mrs. D., a 42-year-old mother of five children, aged 16, 13, 4, 2 years, and 4 months, was hospitalized for the sixth time in 3 years. The father had arranged for a housekeeper through the visiting nurse association and the veterans agency. During the mother's 5 week hospitalization, however, the housekeeper was there only 8 days because she had colds and broke her arm. In addition, the veterans agency would not pay for her services during the children's 1 week vacation from school. The 16-year-old boy (a member of the National Honor Society) and his 13-year-old sister alternated days home from school to care for the three younger children. The 13-year-old girl, however, was absent from school more than her brother "because he hates to miss school and since my marks aren't as good as his, I don't mind it quite as much. I miss my friends though." Except for missing school, these two children stated that they were used to their mother's being away in the hospital. They both had learned how to cook and did not mind caring for the children. The father arrived home from work at 5:30 P.M., but more often than not the 13-year-old had already started to prepare the evening meal. She and her father did the food shopping for the family, and she also helped with the family laundry. With an infant and two other preschool children in the family, this was indeed a major task. After the mother's release from the hospital, both children were able to resume school without further absences; however, after 1 month at home, she pleaded for readmission. This time, she was hospitalized only 8 days and left against medical advice since no plan could be arranged for a housekeeper, no relatives were able to come to the home, and she did not want the children to stay out of school again. Interestingly, the grades of the 13-year-old had improved greatly by the end of the study year because she had had no further absences.

Some older children in two-parent families, with the support of the father in the home after his working hours and the help that the older children gave in the performance of simple household tasks and in the care of the younger siblings after school, allow many families to be maintained without any separations of the children from the home. In the one-parent families, when the older children, 13 to 17 years, did not have the support of the father after his working hours nor a relative in the home, separation of children occurred in two-thirds of the families.

There were nine families that had homemakers for all or part of the time of the mother's hospitalization. In some families one or two children went to live with relatives while others stayed at home and were cared for by a homemaker. Also some families that had previously used relatives' homes for the care of their children had a homemaker, thus preventing further separation of the children from their homes.

Therefore various arrangements were made for child-care when the mothers were hospitalized; they often created serious situations for children whether they were cared for at home or elsewhere. Resources for substitute care were not readily available in most families and there was often delay in placing children.

Care of Children of Ill Fathers

When a father in a family was hospitalized, children generally were cared for by their mothers in their own homes; in these studies there was no separation of children because of the father's hospitalization. In Studies I and II, there were fifty-four hospitalized fathers. In over half of these families the mother was at home, not working, and able to care for the children. In the other 40% of the families, the mother was working regularly to supplement the family income even prior to the father's hospitalization so that the care of the children during the mother's working hours had already been provided for. In one-half of these families, relatives were available to help care for the children in the home until the mother returned from work. In three families, neighbors gave supplementary care, and in the remaining families the mother's working hours coincided with the children's school hours or the children were considered old enough to care for themselves. In only one family with a working mother did the father's hospitalization result in unsatisfactory plans for the care of children.

In this family, the mother had worked regularly from 11:00 P.M. to 7:00 A.M. as a nurse's aide. The father was unemployed for some time prior to his hospital admission and was at home to care for the children during the mother's working hours. When he was hospitalized, their 12-year-old boy stayed home alone during the night with the mother arriving home from work in the morning barely in time to drive him to school. During previous hospitalizations of the father, the boy had to live with relatives since he was younger and the mother could not arrange any other child-care plan. During this hospitalization, she chose to keep him at home and stated that he knew how to use the phone to call the neighbors, the police, the fire department, or the nursing home where she worked (at some distance) should he need any help. The mother stated that she did not like this arrangement for child-care, but she insisted that the boy as well as herself was so accustomed to the father's frequent hospitalizations, they both had learned to get along for these periods without him.

Hospitalization of Children

Some children experienced additional separations when they, themselves, were hospitalized. There were forty-two children from birth through 17 years who were in the hospital at some time during the times of the studies. Almost three-fourths (71%) of these children were 5 years of age or younger. The' reasons for hospitalizations of these children varied: they included six tonsillectomies; a 1-year-old who fell from a carriage (this child was subsequently placed in foster-home care because of question of neglect and abuse); one 8-month child with a skull fracture; eight children in the group of tuberculous patients in Study I hospitalized for tuberculosis, all of whom were 4 years of age or younger; one child 6 weeks of age who died of staphylococcus pneumonia; and two children hospitalized for bronchial conditions.

Separations Due to Mothers' Employment

In addition to the child-care problems presented by hospitalization or incapacity of the mother, there were problems of child-care caused by the mother's employment. At least 34% of the mothers in the three studies were employed immediately prior to or at some time during the study year. Of these 13% were working at both the beginning and end of the study period; 6% were employed at the beginning, but not at the end; 8% began work sometime during the study period and continued in employment at its end; 6.5% worked during a short period only.

The employment of mothers in one-parent families was higher than in two-parent families. Over a third of the mothers were employed sometime during the study year. When fathers were ill, the majority of mothers were employed both at the beginning and end of the study period. Among about half of the mothers employed, the working hours coincided in part with the children's school hours, or the children were old enough to care for themselves. When there were younger children, the mother tried to adjust her working hours to school hours or made some provision for their supervision after school before she arrived home from work with relatives, older children living in the home, or neighbors. Occasionally a child under 12 years of age was left unsupervised during this time.

The most common type of caretaker when the mother was at work were again the grandmothers. They played a major role in 19% of the families in which the mother was employed. In most instances, the grandmothers either lived in the home or came to be with the children while the mother was working. Among 14% of the families in which the mother was employed, the father was the caretaker. In these instances, the mother's employment was in the evening or the husband was at home because of unemployment or illness. Paid caretakers (babysitters) were relied upon in only five instances. In five other cases, at least one child was placed outside the home. In two instances, aunts living in the home or nearby were the caretakers and in another the mother worked part-time as a bookkeeper in her own home. Two mothers worked at night; one left a 12-year-old boy at home alone and the other a 12-year-old boy to care for his siblings. In two families the mothers had left home and were not responsible for their children's care. Thus the mother's employment often resulted in child-care plans, sometimes of questionable adequacy.

Thirty-seven (14.5%) of the total of 253 mothers entered employment sometime during the study year, although they were not working at its beginning. Some worked for financial reasons and others because they enjoyed it.

Following are examples of mothers who started employment during the study year.

Mrs. M. (two-parent) started to work as a nurse's aide about 4 months after discharge from the mental hospital. She worked two nights a week from 3:00 to 11:00 P.M. She claimed that she thoroughly enjoyed the work, and it made her feel useful to others less fortunate than she. She found the extra income helpful and felt that the employment gave her a chance to get away from the household and the children, aged 3 to 15 years. The younger ones were cared for by the two older children and Mr. M. when Mrs. M. was at work. It is noted that Mrs. M. found her 3-year-old son hard to manage.

Mrs. L. (one-parent) started work immediately after discharge from the mental hospital and was employed 6 nights a week as a waitress. She stated that she enjoyed being away from the house as then she did not sit home and worry about her problems. She had been constantly worried about finances because of the irregular contributions from her former husband. Mrs. L. had two older children aged 14 and 8 years, and an illegitimate daughter 9 months of age whom she found hard to handle. She employed a baby sitter to be with the children while she was at work.

Mrs. R. (two-parent), a former mental hospital patient, began to work after she had been brought to court because of complaints that she was neglecting the children. Both the judge and her husband felt that the children should remain temporarily with their paternal grandparents, while Mrs. R. took an outside job, continuing to live alone with her husband. This procedure was followed for a time, but by the year's end Mrs. R. had quit her job and had taken her children back home.

Mrs. O. (two-parent) started to work five evenings a week as a cleaning woman, 1 month after her visit to the Emergency Ward. The family had a history of marital discord and severe financial difficulties, related in part to Mrs. O.'s impulsive spending. She had five children ranging in age from 7 years to 9 months who were cared for by her husband while she was at work. She claimed that she felt better by being able to get out of the house, and her employment seemed to fill a social as well as financial need. Unfortunately, her work did not basically alter the family's indebtedness, which culminated in bankruptcy proceedings at the year's end.

Before Mrs. Y's visit to the Emergency Ward, her husband had not worked for 5 years because of a reported heart condition, and the family was supported by public assistance. Mr. Y. took a job but left it again by the year's end. In the interim, however, Mrs. Y. was employed as a sheet spreader in a laundry and continued to work at the end of the study year. She liked her work and enjoyed the company of the girls she worked with. All of her five children attended school. Mr. Y. assumed responsibility for the household during the day and for the children after school. She reported that the marital friction had lessened since she began to work because she was with her husband less time and was too tired for arguments.

Adequacy of Child Care

The adequacy of the care provided for children when a parent was hospitalized was difficult to determine for several reasons. In the control cases, the decision of adequacy was based in large part on the reports by parents or relatives. In some families, although the care was not ideal, it was considered by relatives and study staff to be the best that was available. The age of the children needing care also influenced the evaluation of adequacy.

In Studies II and III, a method for evaluating the care given by the caretakers was developed. The caretaking function was broken down into four components: time available, health, adequacy, and willingness of the caretaker. Each component was evaluated to see if it was a limiting factor in the adequacy of child-care.

In relation to the component of *time*, any activity inside or outside the home which competed with child-care was considered a limitation. In most cases, such limitations were due to employment. In regard to the factor of *health*, any physical or emotional hendicap which was suggested or implied as interfering with the care of children was considered a limitation. An adequacy limitation was failure of the mother or other responsible caretaker to perform basic care tasks, due to incompetency or lack of "know-how," i.e., ignorance of the duties and responsibilities of motherhood. In rating the component of adequacy in Study II, the emphasis was placed on the physical aspects of caretaking. In Study III, however, where the rating applied only to mothers who were frequently characterized by chronic-type illness and long-term social and emotional deprivation, the inability of the mother to meet normal emotional needs of children was also considered as an *adequacy* limitation. In those cases in Study III in which interpersonal conflict between mother and child was involved, it was frequently difficult to differentiate between limitations associated with the mental or emotional state of the mother and those associated with the inadequate development of her role as mother. In these instances both the health and adequacy components were checked. Finally, the component of *willingness* was checked when there was evidence that the mother or caretaker was unwilling to perform the duties associated with child-care.

In Studies I and II *all* mothers were initially hospitalized so that children were cared for by someone other than the mother, i.e., the father or other caretaker. Thus the ratings in Study II refer to negatives in child-care on the part of one or more substitute caretakers. In Study III, on the other hand, the mother was initially hsopitalized in only a very few cases so that it was she who was rated in relation to her caretaking limitations at the time of the visit to the Emergency Service. The ratings, in the two studies, therefore, are not strictly comparable in the sense that they generally do not refer to the same caretakers (Table 15).

The relatively large proportions of families with *health, adequacy*, and *willingness* negatives in Study III compared with Study II reflect the limitations of the nonhospitalized ill mother who was the person rated in Study III. These proportions were somewhat higher in the two-parent families than in the one-parent families. The difference in the willingness rating between the two studies was less than for the health and adequacy ratings. The large proportion of two-parent families in Study II with *time* negatives is due to the fact that the working father as the responsible caretaker in these families was generally assigned a negative on this component because of his absence

TABLE 15
Families with child-care component negatives—Studies II and III

	Ill parent, study, and number of parents						
	Mother						Father
	Study II (a)			Study III (b)			Study II (a)
Component	Total families (N = 75)	Two (N = 53)	One (N = 22)	Total families (N = 70)	Two (N = 35)	One (N = 35)	(N = 24)
Time	72%	85%	41%	11%	9%	14%	33%
Health	9	6	18	83	91.5	74	0
Adequacy	13	11	18	68.5	71.5	66	4
Willingness	5	2	14	29	20	37	0

(a) Refers to negatives of one or more caretakers.
(b) Refers to negatives of mother only.

during the day. The higher proportions of both two- and one-parent families with ill mothers with negatives in the time component were undoubtedly related to the difficulties of child-care immediately when the mother was hospitalized and to the mother's inadequacy to care for the children when she returned home from the hospital. Finally, the relatively large proportion of families with ill fathers in Study II with a limitation on time (33%) compared to the one-parent families in Study III (14%) is probably the result of the greater number of working mothers in Study II, even though the mother was generally the principal caretaker in both.

More problems in child-care occurred when the mothers were hospitalized or mentally ill than when the fathers were the patients. In Study II almost two-thirds (63%) of families with ill fathers had no child-care problems, while in Study II with ill mothers only 13% of two-parent families and 50% of one-parent families had no child-care problem. There is a striking difference in Study III with ill mothers where only 3% of these urban two-parent families and only 6% of one-parent families had no problems in child-care.

There is also a striking difference in Studies II and III in the number of negatives in child-care. The proportion in Study II of all families with only one negative is much greater than the proportion in Study III. This difference reflects the limitations of the ill mother who was the person rated in Study III, as against other caretakers (usually not the hospitalized mother) rated in Study II. In no family with an ill father, on the other hand, was there more than one negative component.

The following examples illustrate the caretaker situation in families which scored at least two negatives, as seen at the time of the first research interview:

Study II—ill mother

The children in the Y. family (two-parent) were aged 8, 6, and 3 years. The two older children attended school, and Mr. Y. took the 3-year-old to the home of a maternal aunt, who lived in the neighborhood, when he went to work in the morning. The older children returned to the aunt's for lunch and remained there after school until Mr. Y. arrived from work. According to Mr. Y. this caretaking plan had disadvantages, and he was not sure it could continue. The reasons were that the aunt had six children of her own to care for and, in addition, worked a 3:00 to 11:00 P.M. shift in a hospital. Her husband had a heart condition and was unemployed. Mr. Y. feared that the turmoil associated with the presence of so many children would be too much. Mr. Y.'s mother-in-law and her husband lived upstairs in Mr. Y.'s own home. The latter, however, was an alcoholic, and the mother-in-law could not control the children. These in-laws were therefore not available as a caretaking resource. (Negatives on time, health, and willingness.)

The G. family (two-parent) had two children, aged 2 years and 10 months. The 2-year-old son was cared for during the day by a paternal aunt who lived in the same city. Since the aunt was employed at night, Mr. G. picked his son up after work and took him to a maternal aunt in a nearby town for the night. Each morning at 8:00 A.M., he returned him to the first aunt. The youngest child stayed with a second maternal aunt in still another nearby town. This aunt was having a difficult pregnancy, so to relieve her, Mr. G. took his son on weekends to the paternal grandmother, who also lived in the same city as he. (Negatives on time and health.)

Study III—ill mother

Mrs. A. (two-parent) felt nervous, depressed, and cried constantly. She stated that the house felt like a jail and that she had lost her former motivation for cooking and other housework. Shortly before the study year began she had obtained a job in a department store, only to be discharged after a week's work. This had further depressed her. The two children, aged 15 and 17 years, largely cared for themselves. Mrs. A. was described as overly protective and concerned about them. She constantly nagged the 15-year-old son because he was overweight and had no friends or social activities. (Negatives on health, adequacy, and willingness.)

Mrs. P. (one-parent) was described as a hypochondriac, complaining of internal pains and constantly in fear of dying, although no physical basis for the fears or complaints could be found. She was hospitalized for mental illness about 6 months before the beginning of the study year. She left the hospital against medical advice and, together with a daughter 8 years of age, went to live with the maternal grandparents. Two other sons, aged 10 and 11, had been placed with relatives at the time of the mother's hospitalization and continued to live with them. Mrs. P. stated that she had felt too sick to care for her three children since she became ill. The maternal grandmother claimed that Mrs. P. just laid around without participating in housework, cooking, or child-care. She felt that the patient was unconsciously using her illness to avoid caring for her three children. (Negatives on health, adequacy, and willingness.)

In Study II when the ill mother returned to the home at the end of the year, there was a decrease in the proportions of demonstration and control families in which *time* was a negative. There was a corresponding increase in those with a health negative, due to presence in the home of the ill mother. The proportions of families in Study II with negatives on *adequacy* and *willingness* were comparatively small and showed little change. There was a relatively large proportion of families with a *time* negative in which the father was ill which reflected the large proportion of employed mothers in this group. In Study III, there was little change at the end of the study year in the proportion of demonstration and control mothers with ratingngs on any of the four negatives. However, in Study II in the demonstration families, there was a noticeable decrease in the number of families with a negative component *time*, but an increase in those with negative component *health*.

Throughout the case presentations, however, there were frequent indications that whether the children were cared for in their own home, or in a relative's home, was not the sole determining factor in judging the desirability of the child-care arrangements. Families in some instances insisted that the children remain in their own homes, whether or not adequate child-care arrangements were available. On the other hand, some families seemed little concerned about separating their children, not only from their own homes, but perhaps from each other, or from school; and on occasion they were sent to relatives at great distances. One 4-year-old child went to relatives in Trinidad on the day the caretaking relatives learned the mother was to be discharged for they felt she wouldn't be able to care for her child so soon.

Statements in the research interviews with the patient or relatives showed that the duration of the patient's hospitalization had a distinct or direct bearing on the child-care arrangements. The families volunteered frequently that the hospitalization, particularly of the mother, was frankly or perhaps surreptitiously aborted because of her concern about, or dissatisfaction with the care of her children. In addition the mother's concern over the care of her children sometimes influenced the timing of her hospital admission. While some mothers, on admission, had no immediate or expressed concern as to where their children were living or who was caring for them, others, of course, were extremely concerned about the care of their children. They had prepared ahead, as far as they were able, for such tasks as housecleaning, mending, directions for an infant's formula, or food shopping, which made their children more comfortable and their usual care easier to maintain.

These data show convincingly that the child-care problems in families with mentally ill mothers, whether hospitalized or not, created a greater proportion of child-care problems when the families were urban families than if they were families from small cities or suburban areas. This was undoubtedly due to the existence of concurrent problems in these urban families, many of which had existed for some time and which were related to or caused by the mental illness of the mother. These data indicate that these urban families and their children needed assistance from community health and social agencies even before the sick mothers were hospitalized. Because these needs for more adequate child-care occured so often and were so frequently inadequately met, these studies indicate that a planned community approach to this problem is desperately needed.

Summary

A major risk to the children when parents, especially mothers, were hospitalized for mental illness, was caused by their separations from their own homes. For the most part, separations of children were similar whether the mother was hospitalized in a mental hospital or in a tuberculosis sanatorium. When the father in a family was hospitalized, there was relatively little disruption in the living arrangements and care of the children. Disruptions that did occur resulted from the temporary separation of the parents because of marital difficulties ostensibly involved with the father's mental illness prior to his hospital admission. The children in these families with ill fathers continued to live in their own homes, were cared for by their mothers, played with their usual playmates, and continued without interruption in their regular school and play activities. In almost half of the families the mothers were working regularly prior to the fathers' hospitalization, and continued with their employment when the fathers were admitted. Any arrangements for substitute care for the children, because of a mother's employment, were already in effect when the father was hospitalized and, for the most part, continued during her husband's hospitalization to her satisfaction.

When the mother was hospitalized a major factor which determined the risk of separation of children from their own homes was related to the parental composition of the family. When the mothers were hospitalized, children were separated from home in 42% of the families. Factors that largely determined whether or not separation of children occurred were: (1) the availability of relatives for substitute child-care, (2) the ages of the children, and (3) the possibility of paid help or homemaker services. In a third of the families where no separation of children occurred, relatives lived regularly in the home or were willing and able to come to the home to give substitute child-care while in almost a half (46%) the father was able to maintain the care of the children in their own homes. In a few families homemaker services were utilized during the mother's hospitalization, thus preventing separation of children from their homes.

The abruptness of the mother's mental hospitalization, as well as the unknown duration of her stay, complicated the planning for substitute child-care arrangements. Separation of children from home for reasons other than the mother's hospitalization occurred among one-fifth of the families with ill mothers. These other separations were largely a result of the mother's inability to cope with the care of her children even when she was at home. The younger children were more often separated since they required constant supervision and were dependent on the mothers' ability to provide adequate care. Older children, separated for reasons other than the mother's hospitalization, often separated themselves, so to speak, by preferring to live with relatives or friends or, in a few instances, by entering into a precarious marriage to get out of the home.

Relatives provided substitute child-care in their own homes in more than half of the families. However, a substantial proportion, 35%, of families with children separated did not have any consistent child-care plan either for the duration of the first hospitalization or for subsequent admissions. Siblings were often split between realtives. Foster-home placement was used by only a few families. Relatives involved in substitute care of children, whether in the children's own home or not, were sometimes unprepared or unwilling to offer child-care because the time of the mother's hospitalization was inconvenient for them or the repeated requests to care for the children were beginning to dim their tolerance. Their adequacy, willingness, or involvement varied.

In some families it was difficult to decide whether a child was better off staying in his own home during the mother's mental illness or hospitalization or to be cared for away from his own home, thus separating him from not only his own home, but also from siblings, peers, and school. These children had the same risk as other children whose fathers or mothers were absent from the home because of death, divorce, separation, or other reasons, but they also had the added risk of having a parent who was mentally ill for a shorter or longer period of time prior to the hospital admission, and were thereby intimately involved in the disturbances peculiar to mental illness.

About a third of the mothers in the three studies were employed outside the home immediately prior to or some time during the study year. The proportion of employed mothers was slightly higher among one-parent than among two-parent families in Studies I and II and considerably higher among those with ill fathers. Employment of mothers in the urban study, Study III, was somewhat less than in Studies I and II. Slightly over half of the children of employed mothers were of preschool age. The mother worked during school hours, and relied on neighbors, older children, or relatives living in the home to supervise the younger children between he time school closed and her arrival home. Grandmothers and fathers, in that order, served most commonly as substitute caretakers. Fathers were able to fill this role when they themselves were not employed or when their hours of work did not overlap with those of the mother.

The adequacy of the person providing child-care was evaluated at the beginning and end of the study year in Studies II and III in terms of negatives on the four components of *time, health, adequacy,* and *willingness*. The proportion of both two- and one-parent families in Study III with at least two negatives at the year's beginning and end was found to be much greater than in Study II. The difference, however, reflects the limitations of the ill mothers in Study III who were the caretakers and the many problems in social functioning which these families had had for some time.

With the return of the ill mothers from the hospital in Study II, there was an increase in the number of families in which *health* was a negative and a corresponding decrease among those with *time* as a negative. There was little change in Study III with regard to any of the four components in spite of the intensive efforts of the demonstration workers with these families.

7

Efforts to Assist: Community Services

One of the major purposes of the demonstration in both Studies II and III was to develop an effective way of providing to demonstration families services aimed at mitigating or preventing difficulties of children. This section will describe and evaluate the efforts made to provide such services.

The Agencies—Study II

The structure of the demonstration, and therefore the nature of its evaluation, differed in the two studies. In Study II the demonstration was planned as an effort involving a collective responsibility among a group of participating social and health agencies in the community. While the tasks of offering help to the family at the point of crisis and the continuing provision of any needed services were assigned to one agency, it was expected that the services of that agency would be coordinated with those of others in the community so that the principle of community or collective responsibility for the demonstration as a whole would be maintained. The evaluation of the demonstration in Study II, therefore, properly concerns the efforts of all of the participating agencies in the demonstration communities. In contrast, the demonstration staff in Study III were a part of the total study staff and retained the primary responsibility for the provision of social services to study families, as well as for coordinating its efforts with those of other agencies in the community. The fact that the demonstration remained an integral part of the study staff, further-more, made it possible to make a more definitive evaluation of the demonstration effort than could be done in the earlier study.

THE DEMONSTRATION IN STUDY II

Each of the two demonstration communities had acknowledged the importance of mental health problems, although neither of them had previously been involved in any project related primarily to the children of mentally ill parents. One community had a general mental health committee under its council of social agencies and the other had a very active mental health center which had, in the past several years, been working on a community after-care project in conjunction with the state hospital involved in that study. Thus, in each community a climate had been developed for initial acceptance of the demonstration and continued participation in it.

The design of the study called for working agreements between the state hospital and social agencies in the demonstration communities as the hospital social worker needed to know about the patients from a given community and would be serving as a liaison in planning for patients and their children during and after the patient's hospitaliza-tion. In order to do this it was necessary first to identify parents with children at the point of admission, since there was no way of doing this in the usual hospital routine. The agreements were developed during the planning phase of the study, with the project staff taking the lead in joint planning efforts involving the hospital's clinical director and chief of social service and representatives of key agencies in the demonstra-tion communities. At the request of the study staff the hospital admitting office instituted procedures that would produce information, at the time of admission, concerning the presence and ages of children under 18 years of age in the home of the patient. This data proved to be useful to the hospital staff and essential in enlisting the services of agencies in the demonstration communities for child planning.

A family service agency in one community and a mental health center in the second were chosen as "pivot" agencies. Each of these two agencies, in turn, selected a member of its staff to serve as coordinator for the demonstration families. The coordinator from the family service agency was a social worker whose special strength lay in his ability to coordinate the effort of many agencies and other helping persons in the community. However, this agency in the beginning phase had some ambivalence in accepting this responsibility because of its traditional role in the community of working with families who applied for help. Also the Project meant an added burden on the already busy agency. The coordinator from the mental health center was a psychologist. In this community there seemed to be less question as to the leadership role of the center, as well as the eventual integration of the aims of the demonstration into its structure.

The coordinator's role involved making the initial assignment of a demonstration family to an appropriate agency in the community and giving continuity and leadership to the work of the community committee, which are described below. He was also the person in the community who served as a liaison between the community committee and the study staff.

The community committee set up in each of the two demonstration communities was composed of representatives of those agencies whose services were most likely to be needed. Agencies represented on the committees normally included those concerned with public welfare, family service, children's protective services, public schools, public health nursing, as well as a social worker from the state hospital. The representatives from the public schools were guidance personnel, some of whom were social workers. Composition of the committees was kept flexible so as to allow for the addition, during the year, of representatives of agencies potentially helpful to demonstration families. The task of the committees, which met with members of the study staff, was to coordinate over-all community activity on behalf of demonstration families, to influence policy changes where indicated at the local level, and, in general, to maintain and seek to improve the organizational structure for providing services to demonstration families. The committee was also seen as an educational forum where opportunity for joint learning, especially about public health principles, might be provided. The research worker participated actively in setting up and implementing the demonstration committees, as well as in interpreting to the agencies the preventive point of view of the studies. Committees in both communities met on a weekly basis for several months. As the year progressed, however, and working patterns became more routine, the study staff gradually relinquished responsibility to the coordinators in each community, and meetings, unfortunately, were held less frequently.

The agencies in each community agreed to accept the assignment of demonstration families on a rotation basis. They agreed further to make an evaluation of the physical, social, and emotional problems of children in these families, and to provide services as required to the family as a whole in accordance with stated agency function. In accordance with accepted public health procedures, emphasis was placed on intervention at, or as close as possible to, the point of crisis involved in a parent's hospitalization. Agencies were instructed concerning the importance of (1) prompt visit to the family, and (2) continuing support in the form of a reaching-out approach to the family throughout the period of the study. In order to support and maintain these procedures, the study staff made themselves available for frequent conferences with the coordinators and other agency representatives in addition to participating in meetings of community committees. Efforts were also made throughout the year to clarify the working relationships among the study staff, coordinators, and community committees, with emphasis on developing a pattern that the community might find useful for continuing the work of the demonstration after the end of the study.

Problem Areas

Guidelines for agency evaluation of family and children's needs were developed by project staff and distributed to the participating members of the community groups. The guidelines represented a classification of family problems and children's needs. Family problems include those relating to an understanding of the need for or procedures involved in patient's care, marital or parent-child relationships, and financial problems. Children's needs were classified with reference to actual child-care, health supervision, school progress, and emotional adjustment. In addition to the classifications of problems or needs, the guidelines suggested possible ways in which community help might be provided for each type of difficulty.

Three problem areas were considered particularly significant with reference to child-care. These areas concerned housing, income, and caretakers (Table 16). Among the forty demonstration families, there was agency involvement in thirty-one instances. Agencies identified income or financial difficulties in nineteen (61%) of these families, housing difficulites in ten (32%), and caretaker problems in sixteen (52%) others. In nearly all instances agencies made an attempt to provide help with these difficulties. However, the study identified a much larger number of families with problems in each area: income, 81%; housing, 74%; caretaker, 90%.

The nine instances in which there was no agency involvement included those families who had refused agency intervention from the beginning, i.e., at the time when the research interviewer had introduced the idea that someone from the community would be coming to help them. However, these families agreed to participate in the remaining research interviews. From this source and other data

TABLE 16
Demonstration and control families with income, housing and caretaker problems identified by the study, and those identified by one or more community agencies—Study II

| | Type of case and source of data | | | | | |
| | Total Families Active (a) | | Demonstration | | Control | |
Problem area	Study (N = 55)	Agency (N = 55)	Study (N = 31)	Agency (N = 31)	Study (N = 24)	Agency (N = 24)
Income	82%	51%	81%	61%	83%	37%
Housing	71	24	74	52	67	12.5
Caretaker	85.5	44	90	52	79	33
Total study families	99	99	40	40	59	59

(a) With one or more agencies of the seven basic types during the study year.

obtained from school and community agencies, it was learned that at least four of these nine families did have difficulties in one or more of the three areas concerned with income, housing, and caretakers. Refusals to accept community intervention seemed to occur in families of relatively high socio-economic level, in those related to town officials, and in one or two instances in those who were obviously trying to defend themselves from revealing embarrassing marital or personal problems.

The study experience showed that agencies in the demonstration communities were able to commit themselves, in varying degrees, to accepting responsibility for the provision of services to families with a hospitalized parent. In most instances agencies were able to make the immediate home visit suggested by the study, and families generally welcomed it. Participation in the study did involve, however, some problems for agencies. The fact that the agency approached the family as the representative of a community program frequently required a shift in orientation in relation to policy and services, while the focus on children in a preventive frame of reference presented some difficulties even to those agencies that had worked with the mentally ill. Of more immediate concern, however, was the fact that the demonstration did make demands on time and personnel with consequent interruption of the agencies' own schedule of priorities. Even though agencies managed, generally, to honor the inital request for an immediate home visit, the difficulties were reflected in the fact that they frequently were unable to maintain the desired regularity of service through the use of a "reaching-out" type of approach during the study year. It was partly for this reason, of course, that the study staff in Study III was planned so as to include its own demonstration team.

Prior to Study II, communication between the hospital and community agencies was focused primarily at the point of discharge of the patient. The demonstration emphasized the need for social work concern with child-care problems at the point of admission and for the immediate referral of these problems to appropriate community agencies. The demonstration showed that this step not only provided the services needed by the family, but that it also had value to patients who were concerned about their children at home. The participation of the hospital social worker in the community meetings facilitated communication between hospital and community and, in fact, symbolized the hospital's participation as part of the community. Communication was also furthered by patient conferences concerned largely with after-care planning which were held at the hospital and to which community representatives were invited.

Demonstration—Study III

It was possible to carry out an evaluation of the demonstration effort for each of the thirty-five demonstration families in Study III at the end of the study year. Data available concerning the demonstration in Study III is therefore more detailed and exhaustive than was true in Study II. The evaluation was concerned with the following aspects of the demonstration: (1) problem areas of the family as seen by the demonstration worker; (2) involvement of the demonstration worker in relation to specific problems; (3) movement of the family during the year in relation to these problems; (4) the association between the worker's involvement and movement; (5) community agencies contacted by the demonstration workers; (6) purpose of such contacts; (7) effectiveness of community resources; and (8) maintenance of contacts by agencies to whom families were referred, following the end of the demonstration year. These factors are described in detail below.

Problem Areas

Difficulties in family functioning were rated in relation to twenty problem areas (Table 17). These areas were grouped so that five related primarily to the patient, three to the father, three to the family as a whole, two to the environment, and seven to one or more children in the family. The number of demonstration families with difficulties in each of the twenty problem areas some time during the year was noted by the raters. The raters were three demonstration social workers plus two social workers employed only for rating the material. Each rater scored separately and independently. The results were pooled and a final judgment was arrived at by agreement with all raters. Problems were checked as applying at two points in time, the beginning and the end of the demonstration year. The data in the table, however, refer to difficulties noted at either or both of these times. The rating was made on the basis of any difficulty, one or more, that pertained to any given problem area. Many of these difficulties were chronic and persistent in nature, and all except very minor and transient difficulties were included.

The basis of the rating in a few of these problem areas needs additional explanation. The area involving the mother as a child caretaker includes not only physical caretaking, which is the provision of the children's material needs, but also the emotional quality of mothering, and parent-child relationships. Among the seven problem areas involving children, any difficulty that concerned one child was rated for the area as a whole even though it did not apply to the other children in the family.

In regard to the mother as the child caretaker, her ability to meet the child's needs was sometimes judged in relation to her mode of interaction with the child or to physical, social, or behavioral problems of the child in which the involvement of the mother was known or assumed. Thus, if the mother was not following recommendations of the pediatrician, she was rated as having a problem in child-care. Physically neglected and ill-fed children were seen as evidence of the mother having a problem in this area.

TABLE 17
Problem areas during year as rated by the
demonstration by number of parents

Problem area (a)	Total	Number of parents	
		Two-parent	One-parent
Patient			
Health	26	14	12
Mental or emotional	35	19	16
As child caretaker	35	19	16
As homemaker	17	7	10
Employment	12	4	8
Father			
Health (b)	19	13	6
Father-child relationship	18	11	7
Employment	14	11	3
Family			
Marital situation	26	16	10
Relationship with relatives	25	14	11
Leisure-recreation	29	16	13
Environmental			
Housing or neighborhood	28	14	14
Finances	32	17	15
Total families	35	19	16
Health	87	46	41
Neurotic traits	41	28	13
Behavior	40	18	22
School	46	25	21
Retardation	2	1	1
Sib relations	29	16	13
Peer relations	32	17	15
Total children	103	54	49

(a) Noted at the beginning and/or end of the study year.
(b) Includes mental and physical health.

The psychological capacity of the mother to mother was more difficult to judge, since it required an assessment on the part of the demonstration worker that the mother could not meet the child's emotional needs. In some instances, mothers could not meet their children's insistent demands for mothering, and rejection of the child was evident. In others a real struggle in the mother-child relationship could be observed. In other cases, however, mothers, whose psychic energy was used up in their own intrapersonal conflicts, had little left for their children or were psychologically unavailable to them. In still other cases mothers literally did not possess the "know-how" in relation to their responsibilities in child-care and homemaking tasks. It was not uncommon for mothers to look to the demonstration worker for helpful hints, and often were grateful when the demonstration worker suggested how a situation might be handled, or how they could relate to their husbands or children in a more satisfying manner.

The health problems of children were rated on the basis of the first report of the examining pediatrician, as well as the demonstration worker's knowledge gained through a year of contact with the family and community. Failure to complete immunizations, obtain health supervision as needed, or to provide medical or dental follow-up services for any health symptom or condition was rated as a health problem. Parents frequently did not seem to understand the concept of preventive care, and it was difficult for them to respond to this need even when pressure was brought to bear. For example, one mother seemed unable to finish her 2-year-old child's immunizations, even though she lived only half a mile from the Child Health Chinic and passed it frequently to shop or visit a friend.

Some of the problems were much more frequent than others among the thirty-five families and 103 children. The most frequent problem areas noted were the patient's health, the patient's mental or emotional condition, the patient as child caretaker, the marital situation, relations with relatives, leisure-time recreation, housing or neighborhood, finances, and children's health. The prevalence of the latter difficulty, however, reflected the inclusion of the need for health supervision in the rating. Other problem areas of children less frequently noted were those involving school difficulties, overt behavior difficulties, and those that were primarily psychoneurotic in nature.

The proportions of one- and two-parent families with many of these problem areas were similar. Obviously, those areas relating to the father, including the marital situation, were underrrepresented among the one-parent families. The one-parent families, however, did show an excess of problems involving the mother as a homemaker, as well as those concerning the mother's employment. The following are examples.

(1) Patient's employment

Mrs. T. (one-parent) was an intelligent woman and in her more rational moments quite responsible in her employment. Actually it was the only strength she had and the only area where she could function well. However, due to adolescent interests, she did not like to work during the summer, preferring to draw unemployment insurance benefits while talking about how difficult it was to find a job.

She became conniving and manipulative in this area, as in all others. She would find jobs with "shady" people or outfits, leaving herself open to difficulties with the law. Rather than working, she would think it quite clever "to find" clients for her friends who were lawyers or insurance men—accepting a "kickback."

This girl was a willful, narcissistic, immature, young woman. She did what she wanted, when she wanted. When she felt like it, she returned to work and did an excellent job, taking a good deal of responsibility in an office and receiving a raise.

(2) Patient as homemaker

Mrs. M's (one-parent) total life was disorganized and inadequate. The problem seemed to stem from two sources, her depression and lack of homemaking ability. The home was described by the demonstration worker as chaotic and dirty. After considerable persuasion from the demonstration worker, the _____ Association agreed to provide a homemaker for this difficult mother. Patient was able to accept this service and use it appropriately.

There was, surprisingly, a smaller number of children with neurotic type problems in one-parent compared to two-parent families (X^2 = 5.5, P < .05), although this was somewhat counterbalanced by an excess of children with problems involving overt behavior difficulties (not significant). A further breakdown of the data on neurotic problems showed that these differences were maintained for all age groups.

(1) Children with neurotic problems

Mrs. C. (one-parent), a woman still very dependent on her parental family, had considerable trouble because of the excessive dependence of her own four children, aged 14, 9, 7, and 4 years. It was very difficult to handle these problems with the mother because of her own involvement in this area. All children were described by the school as withdrawn, depressed, sad, and immature. One child had a sleep distrubance and anxiety. An arranged camp experience for the children was very difficult as both mother and children had a difficult time separating. Therefore, the children were hard to manage at camp and did not enjoy the experience.

(2) Children with behavior problems

The T. children (one-parent) were hyperactive, demanding, immature, unmanageable, and continually seeking attention. The oldest boy, age 9, however, was the most affected by the family tensions. His whole life had been spent in a home with severe marital problems, and eventual divorce of his parents. He had suffered the most from the lack of mothering. All family members blamed him for parents' ill-fated marriage. With this background he was a most unappealing child. He suffered particularly by comparison with his younger brother, the favored child, who was much more likeable. H., the oldest child, was used as a barometer of the household tensions. It was clear that when H. was cooperative, the total family was not under undue stress.

TABLE 18
Number of children with problems by age and sex

| | | Age in years, and sex | | | | | | | |
| | Total | 0-2 | | 3-5 | | 6-12 | | 13-17 | |
Problem area	children	M	F	M	F	M	F	M	F
Health	87	10	10	11	8	25	14	5	4
Neurotic traits	41	4	2	4	5	12	9	3	2
Behavior	40	3	1	5	3	16	4	6	2
School	46	–	–	3	3	19	11	7	3
Retardation	2	1	0	0	0	1	0	0	0
Sibling relations	29	2	1	5	2	6	7	4	2
Peer relations	32	3	0	1	3	12	3	7	3
Total children	103	11	13	15	11	26	14	9	4

The children's problems were further broken down by age and sex (Table 18). Problems of physical health were predominant in children at all ages. Problems involving behavior and peer relations were especially predominant in the teenage group whereas school problems were found among the great majority of school age children. The problems were, in general, evenly distributed between the sexes in the several age groups. However, a larger proportion of girls than of boys ages 6-12 years had sibling problems, while the proportion of girls in the 0-2 year group was smaller than that of boys for all types of difficulties.

(1) Children with health problems (aged 0-2)

Mrs. T. (one-parent) was immediately interested in the study's offer of a pediatric examination. Perhaps this may have been the chief factor in giving the demonstration worker an entré as Mrs. T., who had known many social workers and psychiatrists in the past, felt that no one was really interested nor was going to help. E., age 1 year, was seen at the _____ Hospital for nutritional problems and speech difficulties. The frenum was clipped, but there was no follow-through for speech therapy. In regard to speech therapy and nutritional follow-up, the doctor was quoted as saying, "We have no time for well children; she looks all right to me."

Mrs. T. responded well to the study's pediatric recommendations and was initially ready and able to follow through on them. However, her intital experiences at the _____ Hospital were dissatisfying in spite of her continued efforts to obtain treatment for her children. Throughout the year, even with the two older children, she was subject to differing medical opinions between her private doctor and the outpatient departments of two hospitals. This was particularly noticeable in the mother's trying to follow through on a T & A. By the end of the year she was so discouraged that she intitally refused the final pediatric examination of the study, feeling it was all useless. Eventually, however, she agreed to the examination

The C. family (two-parent) lived on a marginal income, but spent a large proportion—about 10%—on medical expenses. The family used a number of doctors and dentists in their area, but somehow chronic health problems of the children did not improve. Two children had ear difficulties. When the study pediatrician and the school both suggested that one child might have a hearing loss, the mother denied this, insisting that her own physician would have diagnosed this. Another child had had an eye operation at least 5 years previously. Although eyeglasses were recommended, the teenage boy involved was not interested, and the mother saw no reason for pursuing the matter further.

This family was resistant to the recommendations of the study pediatrician that the child go to the outpatient department of a general hospital nearby. Although the demonstration worker arranged for a reduced fee at the hospital and persuaded the mother to have the children seen there once, there was a strong indication that the family would not continue to use this available facility after the study year.

(2) Children with school problems (aged 6-12)

Mrs. O. (one-parent) had four children, three of whom were in parochial school at the time of the first contact. M., a 9-year-old girl, was withdrawn and, as judged by the school, was not working up to her potential ability. E., aged 10, was described as lackadaisical and a daydreamer. He was found by the school clinic to have a visual difficulty, and glasses were prescribed. However, the study pediatrician reported that he did not wear them. E. had a reading problem, and his school work was considered to be at a level below that of his real ability. He did, however, receive tutoring during the year. Both children were seen as emotionally disturbed by the demonstration. In the opinion of the school authorities, the school problems were associated with their relationship with their parents.

(3) Child with a peer relationship problem

D.D., age 16 (one-parent family), had been an aggressive, acting-out boy for some years, often on the fringe of delinquent activities. He came from a neighborhood where men are notorious for making their living through "shady" and delinquent activities.

At age 14, this boy attacked and killed his father during a family quarrel and was in a training school for a year. He then returned home, but his parole was revoked shortly thereafter as his mother was unable to manage him. After 2 more years in a training school, D. became a hero in his neighborhood, a leader of the delinquent boys. He was looked up to and held in high esteem for having killed his father. This image was an uncomfortable position for the boy. He was not particularly bright, and perhaps not of average intelligence. He did not see himself as a leader and did not want the responsibility, even though he was enchanted with the status. The possibility of arranging more comfortable and appropriate peer relationships for this child was extremely difficult and perhaps impossible, as he was continually sought after by the youngsters and adults as a leader.

Among the thirty-five demonstration families, all but two were rated as having difficulties in ten or more of the twenty possible problem areas. Twenty or 57.1% had problems in fifteen or more types, and the thirteen remaining families had problems in from ten to fourteen types. The one- and two-parent families did not differ with respect to the multiplicity of types of problems. The following two examples describe families with multiple problems.

1) The parents in the T. family (two-parent) were a young couple in their early twenties. Both had been reared in disorganized, inadequate families. Throughout their marital history the husband had shown difficulties in relating to the patient. He regularly left the patient for about 6 months of the year, during which time he would drive around the New England area.

Though these two people brought little to their marriage, one might assume that they could have lived a marginal life had they had no major difficulties. However, after almost 2 years of marriage, their twin daughter died. Neither parent had the maturity or strength to face the death of their baby nor had they a realtionship together which could help them face and work out their grief. The death of this child is central to nearly all problem areas with this family.

The father left the family for 7 months of the demonstration year, so that he was less well-known to the demonstration worker than other members of the family. He requested help and knew he needed it in the following areas: mental health, the father-child relationship, the marital situation, housing, income, employment, and leisure-recreation. Emotionally he was unable to face the problems and use the help that could be given. He seemed to prefer a man to relate to, and perhaps would have responded well to a male social worker. However, the father returned to the home at the end of the year, having resolved his marital and employment difficulties in an unusual way. He had a good job with the post office and worked at sorting mail. This, of course, provided an adequate income and took him away from his family for a part of each week, which gave him the relief he needed in the marital situation.

Mother's emotional problems added to her difficulties in many areas. She was unable to seek proper health supervision for herself or her child; her ability as a child caretaker was severely limited; her marriage was poor; she was socially isolated, a condition that was related to her leisure and housing difficulties. The tie-in with her central problem was interesting. She found herself to be helpless in the face of maternal grandmother's "crazy" behavior and frightened of having everyone witness it, as they would then ridicule mother. Mother had learned that when she tried to make friends the maternal grandmother would interject herself into the relationship in such a way as to alienate mother's friends. Mother handled this by living in isolated neighborhoods, which cut her and her child off from any social relationships.

The reaction of the living twin to the twin's death would have to be seen in terms of the developmental tasks for his age. As each developmental task was impaired by mother's withdrawal and inability to help with the task, the task was not completed well or within a healthy setting, therefore adding another layer to and broadening the family's difficulties. At age 2 months basic mothering was withheld due to the separation of parents and the subsequent poor living arrangements, coupled with mother's withdrawal in response to her grief. As time went on, mother then was unable to find a toehold with which to break the cycle. At the time of inital contact of the demonstration worker, the problem had grown and was found in a severe feeding problem. Mother was unable to face her child without extreme tension. Feeding was done then in an abrupt tense manner. The child quickly picked up mother's tension and preoccupation, and either refused food or vomited what was eaten.

2) The parents in the N. family (two-parent) were in their early forties and had seven children ranging in age from 19 to an infant born approximately 9 months after the initial contact. The patient reported that there had always been marital discord, which had become progressively worse with the years. Father's drinking and abuse of mother and children had been problems. Although father had 2 years of schooling after high school, he was satisfied with a mediocre job which did not employ his skills. It had been necessary for mother to work for the past 10 years to meet debts. In addition, Mr. N. was unrealistic in his expectations of the mother's ability to manage on the money which he provided. The mother frequently had to obtain additional money from the maternal grandmother.

The patient was hospitalized the day following her appearance at the emergency service with a diagnosis of acute schizophrenia. Although she was subsequently released from the hospital, there were two further hospitalizations during the year, one a suicidal attempt resulting in a coma. On this occasion the father visited in the hospital and assaulted the mother.

During the time that she was at home there was a serious question about the patient's capacity to mother because of her narcissism and projection patterns. She had little ability to comprehend the needs of her children, could not be flexible and giving to the baby, and did not feed him enough. She related to the children in an inconsistent, possessive way. She had no friends of her own and indicated that she felt uncomfortable in bringing anyone home because of the husband's drinking.

The effect of the emotional and marital problems in this family had left their mark on the children. The 19-year-old daughter left school in the tenth grade to work and help the family. She married just prior to the initial contact and left for California with an immature and irresponsible husband. Within the year she was contemplating separation. The next two children completed high school. One, a girl, felt some responsibility for the home and was overburdened with the care of the family during mother's hospitalizations. The second, a boy, hoped to attend college, was angry and bitter, and isolated himself from the family. A seventh grade boy had repeated several grades and had a reading problem.

The father denied his problems and would not use help. Mother was unable to follow through unless there was aggressive reaching out. Even then it was difficult for the worker to get through mother's denial and hostility.

Involvement of Demonstration Worker—Study III

The thirty-five demonstration families were individually rated in relation to the extent of involvement of the demonstration worker with each of the twenty problem areas during the year (Table 19). Extent of involvement in any given problem was rated relative to that in all problems and was classified into four groups: minimal, moderate, extensive, and none. The demonstration workers were involved in some way in the great majority or existing problems relating to the patient, father, family as a whole, and the environment. However, the workers were involved somewhat less frequently in the problem areas relating to children. Among the areas in which the worker was involved, furthermore, the extent of the involvement in individual problem areas affecting children was reduced when compared to the attention that she gave to other problems affecting the adults and family as a whole. Most of her involvements with children's problems were minimal in extent, whereas a much larger proportion of her involvements with other types of problems were moderate or extensive. The latter is true in those areas involving the patient and the family as a whole, as well as in areas of finances and the father's employment.

The lesser involvement with children's problems was not by design, but reflects the resistance and other difficulties encountered by the demonstration worker when she attempted to explore these areas. In part this seemed to be due to the severity of the patient's own problems which had to be dealt with before involvement could be attained in other areas. In part this seemed also the result of defensiveness on the patient's part about the worker's role with her children. The following brief accounts illustrate the difficulties faced by the caseworker in attempting to deal with problems of children.

1) Mrs. F. (two-parent) had had two long mental hospitalizations in the past. She was a severely disturbed woman and an alcoholic. It was presumed that she was sexually promiscuous with both men and women. She would leave her home before 7:30 A.M. and sometimes stayed away for days. Father worked, and the 12-year-old boy had the main care of the younger children, aged 10 and 8.

The major problem in this case was in making contact with both, or either, parent. The demonstration worker had more contact with father throughout the year than mother. His main interest was in trying to get mother hospitalized, if only for her own protection. He felt he could take care of the children. Therefore, he enlisted the worker's help mainly in the hospitalization procedure.

One can presume that it would have taken father a long time to accept and work on his children's problems, even if he had the time and motivation. However, his time at least was spent working to support the children. The worker did manage to make contact with the children in some areas but it is extraordinarily difficult to bring help to children when contact cannot be made with the parents.

2) Mrs. M. (one-parent) had been hospitalized at the beginning of the year and her own problems subsequent to this were so severe that the worker did not have the opportunity to deal extensively with those of her six children. Thus, lack of involvement in the children's problems was not due to the mother's obstruction, but to the priorities of the case. The mother, in fact, seemed to welcome the help she did receive in relation to the children; especially a 6-year-old son, who was stealing and acting out in what seemed to be a reaction to the recent loss of his father, was referred by the demonstration worker to an outpatient psychiatric unit where he was seen for a diagnostic evaluation. The patient accepted this referral and cooperated with it.

In general, however, it was difficult to cover many different problems with a hard-to-reach, crisis-ridden family. The primary time-consuming concern here was simply to assure the physical care of the children. This meant that once the patient had returned from the hospital a good deal of time had to be spent keeping her on her feet.

3) Mrs. T. (one-parent) and maternal grandmother (chief caretaker) were unable to face the children's problems and provide solutions.

TABLE 19
Type of problem and extent of involvement of demonstration worker

Type of Problem	Total cases with problem noted	DW not involved	Total with involvement	Extent of demonstration worker's involvement (a)		
				Minimal	Moderate	Extensive
Patient						
Health	26	5	21	11	3	7
Mental or emotional	35	1	34	5	8	21
As child caretaker	35	6	29	8	13	8
As homemaker	17	6	11	6	2	1
Employment	12	0	12	5	6	1
Father						
Health	19	7	12	6	4	2
Father-child relations	18	6	12	11	1	0
Employment	14	3	11	8	2	1
Family						
Marital situation	26	2	24	5	8	11
Relations with relatives	25	3	22	14	4	4
Leisure-recreation	29	5	24	13	6	5

Environment						
Housing or neighborhood	28	5	23	18	3	2
Finances	32	5 (b)	27	14	11	2
Total families	35	35	35	35	35	35
Health	87	34	53	39	7	7
Neurotic traits	41	20	21	16	2	3
Behavior	40	14	26	16	6	4
School	46	25	21	20	0	1
Retardation	2	1	1	0	0	1
Sib relations	29	16	13	10	1	1
Peer relations	32	18	14	12	0	2
Total children	103	103	103	103	103	103

(a) Extent of involvement in any given problem is rated relative to that in all problems.
(b) Includes one case where problem was noted, but the involvement was rated as unknown.

Rather than facing the crucial issues, they would settle on a minor or unrealistic problem and become concerned about it. For example, the children were unmanageable in the home, particularly when mother was acting out. Mother and maternal grandmother denied the children's uncontrollable behavior, but became involved in the fact that H. received a poor mark in handwriting and needed tutoring in this subject. To have faced the children's problems would have meant to face their own problems. This they could not do. They did not want any help in understanding that the children were reacting to the adults' neurotic behavior. Maternal grandmother could consider mother's responsibility, but neither could face their own relationship with the children and the effect it was having. When efforts were made by the worker to help them face this issue, they would say they were not ready, would deny the problem, and report that the children did not need any help. Their anxiety became heightened when the suggestion of introducing a Big Brother was made.

Social Work Treatment

The supportive casework technique was the one primarily used by the demonstration workers in working with study families. In a few instances this technique was, however, combined with reflective discussion and/or confrontation. Reflective discussion, a technique described by Hollis (1964), is concerned with helping the client understand the reasons for, or the consequences of, his behavior, especially when it is influenced by distorted perceptions or lack of knowledge. Confrontation, as described in a report of the Community Service Society (1958) "consists of pointing out sterotyped or patterned episodes in the client's behavior, attitudes or feelings which he needs to become aware of, and can tolerate awareness of, in order to improve his functioning." These techniques are sometimes hard to differentiate in practice, and the following two examples illustrate elements of either or both.

1) Mrs. H. (one-parent) expressed her rejection of her 6-year-old daughter, W., and her wish that W. would die, tieing this in with the

fact that she had been told immediately after birth that W. was dead. Mother saw W. as probably the major reason for her emotional difficulties and wondered why W. had not been killed under the beatings and treatment that she had given her. She was relieved when the demonstration worker questioned this and interpreted it as her way of asking for W.'s placement outside of the home.

The worker confronted Mrs. H. directly with the relationship between her feelings about W., her inability to make a decision regarding her marital situation, and her need for psychiatric treatment. Mrs. H. agreed to cooperate with placement plans. Through reflective discussion she was also able to face the fact that much of W.'s behavior was in direct reaction to the way that mother treated W. Although W. often acted out with others, when with mother she answered everything, "Yes ma'am, No ma'am," When the demonstration worker wondered why this might be, mother readily responded by accepting the fact that W. was frightened of her.

2) Mrs. Y.'s (two-parent) 16-year-old daughter "runs away." When found, parents "beat" her, and she subsequently ran away again. This process was readily described by the mother to the demonstration worker who questioned the method of handling this situation by the parents. The demonstration worker's response initally brought agitation and anger. Later in the interview. however, mother was able to calm down and face with the demonstration worker how worried and frightened she was when she could not find her daughter; her daughter's reaction to the beating; and her own reaction when she had been beaten at age 16.

Some form of environmental manipulation was used with about 70% of the families. Direct advice or guidance was increasingly given by the demonstration workers as the year went on. Two examples of the workers' activities in providing direct advice or guidance and environmental manipulation are given below.

(1) Direct advice or guidance

In working with the U. family (two-parent), the worker had to use the techniques of direct advice or guidance extensively because of the severe intellectual and cultural inadequacies of the parents.

Once a relationship had been built, it was important to them to be able to use the demonstration worker's advice to report the results the next week. Direct advice and constant direction were used in all health matters. The demonstration worker checked every week on how much medication mother had and would tell her when to return to the psychiatric service for more.

The demonstration worker tried to help mother and child separate, in order that child should spend less time with parents and more time in the community. Mother was unable to allow her 13-year-old son to go anywhere alone. Considerable time was spent in planning a program with the Boys' Club. However, mother at first would walk the child to the club and return early to wait for him. With very definite guidance the demonstration worker helped mother to stop this practice and suggested she at least wait at the corner most distant from the club. Eventually this worked, and on occasion the child was allowed to travel to and from the club without mother.

In addition to the above areas, the demonstration worker at times gave specific directions regarding the feeding of the child and family, cleanliness of the child, cleaning the home, budgeting, and buying. Definite limits were set on inappropriate buying. This technique was used to an exceptional degree with this family because the more usual supportive techniques were not effective. It worked best in separating the mother and child, but even then was painfully slow. It also worked reasonably well in keeping the mother on her medication. It did not, however, work in all areas. The parents, for instance, would not always report their spending once they knew the demonstration worker's stand on the issue.

(2) Guidance and environmental manipulation

In the T. family (two-parent) guidance and environmental manipulation were used in relation to the patient's mental health, the mother role, finances, and leisure-recreation. The demonstration worker spent considerable time making contact with various agencies that were concerned with Near-Eastern people (family was Armenian), particularly in regard to leisure-recreation. Through the worker's advice and guidance mother was able to use these agencies in order to break her isolation.

The demonstration worker helped mother obtain extra financial assistance for her tranquilizers and contraceptive pills. With the worker's guidance she was even able to consider using the Syrian-

Lebanese Child Welfare Society for camp. This was an unusual achievement, due to mother's strong feelings *against* any type of "welfare."

Movement in the Problems

While many difficulites rated by the demonstration at the beginning of the year remained at the end, they did not necessarily remain at the same intensity. That is, it would be expected that some problems became less acute, whereas others did not change or became worse. Each family was evaluated with regard to movement shown during the year for each of the problem areas noted at the beginning of the year. For each of these problem areas one out of five movement ratings was given: extensive improvement, moderate improvement, minimal im provement, no change, or deterioration.

The movement of families with regard to each of the twenty individual problem areas was analyzed (Table 20). Although some improvement was noted in every area, gains were particularly noticeable in those involving the patient's mental or emotional health, her role as a child caretaker, father's employment, leisure-recreation, housing or neighborhood, and the children's physical health. In those instances in which improvement did occur it was most frequently rated moderate or extensive, as opposed to minimal, in the patient's role as homemaker, the father's employment, housing, and in the children's school problems. Other problem areas in which substantial improvement was achieved, although less frequently, included the patient's mental or emotional health, leisure-recreation, the financial situation, and children's health. Illustrations of minimal, moderate, and extensive improvement in one area, that of the mother as a homemaker, are given below. With this as an example of the range of improvement during a year, examples of gains in other areas are limited to those with ratings of moderate improvement.

TABLE 20
Movement rating for problems noted at beginning of year

	Total with problem at beginning	Unable to rate	No change	Deteri-oration	Total improved	Mini-mal	Mod-erate	Exten-sive
						Degree of improvement		
Patient								
Health	25	6	11	0	8	5	1	2
Mental or emotional	35	1	11	4	19	10	8	1
As child caretaker (a)	34	5 (b)	11	3	15	10 (c)	4 (c)	1 (c)
As homemaker	17	0	9	2	6	2	3	1
Employment	7	0	5	0	2	1	0	1
Father								
Health	18	5	9	2	2	2	0	0
Father-child relations	18	2	12	2	2	2	0	0
Employment	12	1	5	1	5	2	2	1
Family								
Marital situation	25	3	11	3	8	5	3	0
Relations with relatives	19	0	11	2	6	3	2	1
Leisure-recreation	26	0	13	1	12	6	6	0

Environmental								
Housing or neighborhood	27	1	16	0	10	3	5	2
Finances	32	3	17	1	11	6	3	2
Total families	35	35	35	35	35	35	35	35
Health	75	8	35	1	31	18	11	2
Neurotic traits	32	6	17	1	8	6	1	1
Behavior	35	3	17	6	9	7	2	0
School	34	6	20	1	7	2	4	1
Retardation	2	1	1	0	0	0	0	0
Sib relations	23	0	17	0	6	5	1	0
Peer relations	24	5	13	2	4	2	1	1
Total children	103	103	103	103	103	103	103	103

(a) A combined rating of mother's ability to mother, her ability as a physical caretaker, and her relationship with individual children.

(b) Includes three families, in each of which an improvement in one of the items comprising this rating is balanced by deterioration in another.

(c) Rating indicated is the highest of each of the three separate ratings comprising this problem area.

(1) Mother as homemaker—minimal improvement

Mrs. Y. (one-parent) had been hospitalized briefly at the beginning of the demonstration, following a serious suicide attempt, and returned home while still in a deteriorated state. She and her two children lived in crowded conditions with the maternal grandparents. Emotionally Mrs. T. was rebellious and demanding and seemed in need of controls. The grandparents were unable to supply these controls for their adult child and were, furthermore, afraid of relating to her at all for fear of precipitating another suicidal attempt. Mother, a master manipulator, made good use of her parents' inability to control her and refused to take any part in the running of the household or the care of her children.

Toward the end of the year, however, during which time she had fully cooperated in social casework treatment at the _____ Hospital, she began to take minimal responsibility in the home. At the same time the demonstration worker strongly supported the grandmother, who herself had a heart condition, but feared placing any demands on the mother in allowing the latter to take over some of the homemaking tasks. By the year's end she was able to make her bed in the morning before leaving for work, keep her room picked up in accordance with minimal standards, and to offer the grandmother minimal help in spring housecleaning. She had also begun to talk about setting up her own apartment for herself and children.

(2) Mother as homemaker—moderate improvement

Mrs. N. (two-parent) complained initially at length about her inability to care for the home without considerable help from children and father. This was not seen to be a problem by the demonstration worker, who felt that the expectations of this Italian mother may have been, in part, culturally determined. The possibility that she might not normally require children to do their part would only increase her discomfort in a situation in which the demonstration worker realistically felt that they should take on certain responsibilities in the home.

By the end of the year the mother's complaints had stopped, and she was carrying on her homemaking tasks with ease. Improvement in this case was rated on the change in the attitude and complaints of the mother rather than on a change in her actual homemaking ability.

(3) Mother as homemaker—extensive improvement

At the initial interview with the demonstration worker Mrs. E. (two-parent) verbalized homemeker difficulties as one of the reasons for her emotionally upset condition. She claimed to be a compulsive housekeeper and noted that she was unable to tolerate even minimal disorganization, even when there might be a realistic reason for it. The fact that Mr. E. was currently helping her in the home was seen as a negative by Mrs. E., supporting her poor self-image and fear that she could not function.

The demonstration worker's involvement in this problem area was limited to supporting the mother by praising her homemaking skills, as well as providing some advice and guidance. By the end of the year, however, the mother was again able to cope with her homemaking tasks in accordance with her own standards. In addition, she was able to find time to leave the home, join groups, and obtain a part-time job.

(4) Father's employment—moderate improvement

At the beginning of the year Mr. C. (two-parent) had two jobs (9:00 A.M.-4:00 P.M.; 9:00 P.M.-4:00A.M.). This caused problems in the marriage and with father-child relationships, as father basically was not in the home. It also left the father little time for sleep.

By the end of the year the family had caught up on bills, and he gave up the evening job. This brought about an immediate improvement in the marriage. The mother became pregnant, which seemed to satisfy the needs of both parents.

The change in the employment situation was thus not only favorable in itself for the father, but it had an effect on other family difficulties and satisfied needs of other family members.

(5) Mother's mental health—moderate improvement

Mrs. R. (one-parent) was hospitalized within a week after initial contact. She remained at _____ State Hospital for about a week and was returned home. In less than a week mother voluntarily returned to the hospital again where she remained for approximately a month, returning home with the plan that she would continue her psychiatric therapy through _____ State Hospital's psychiatric outpatient deparment. This plan was never realized, partly because of realistic transportation problems. At the time of the initial hospitalization mother was in poor mental health, being very depressed and having made a suicidal gesture.

The movement in this case had little, if anything, to do with any psychiatric treatment that mother received, whether from the State Hospital or the demonstration worker. The mother was unable to relate and use help. She was unable to face her problems in any way but a superficial, cursory manner. Her breakdown seemed mainly to be caused by the birth of her daughter born out-of-wedlock. Once her father stopped verbally rejecting her and they began to correspond, mother again returned to marginal functioning. If she did not suffer a major rejection from anyone and were allowed to remain quite dependent upon her family, mother's prognosis seemed good, and it appeared possible she would never be hospitalized again.

Mother received a moderate rating because she was out of the hospital at the end of the year, had been out for approximately 9 months, and showed no signs of deterioration. Her general functioning was adequate.

(6) Leisure-recreation—moderate improvement

A good deal of Mrs. T.'s (one-parent) acting out was seen in this area. She sought only leisure, and then would behave inappropriately. As if in adolescent rebellion, she would seek out only the "shadier" spots in town to attend, enjoying the criminal and delinquent element. She was promiscuous. By the end of the year she was able to stay at home occasionally without fulfilling the almost compulsive need to leave her home and family. On occasion she would get together with her girl friends. She obtained a part-time evening job in which she sold cosmetics at ladies' clubs. She began to find enjoyment and fulfillment in leisure and recreation which was not potentially destructive to herself.

(7) Children's health—moderate improvement

With the help of Operation Headstart, the M. family (one-parent) was referred to the _____ Hospital Family Health Clinic. This clinic offered comprehensive medical and social services, utilizing a reaching-out approach. Although the mother continued to be somewhat remiss in following through on appointments and recommendations, the fact that this referral was successfully made indicated moderate improvement in this area. The demonstration worker encouraged follow-through by supporting the mother with advice and guidance, and by maintaining contact with the clinic regarding this family.

Movement and Mothers' Involvement

The distribution of the movement ratings in each of the twenty problem areas for those families and children with which the demonstration workers were minimally or not involved, and moderately or extensively involved, is shown in Table 21. The involvement of the worker in some of the problem areas is associated with improvement. This is seen most strongly in the area of children's health. Eleven or 78.6% of the fourteen children with health problems in which the worker was moderately or extensively involved improved, as compared to only twenty or 37.7% of the fifty-three children whose health problems could be rated and in which the worker was minimally or not involved (X^2 = 5.8, P < .05). A similar association, which just misses significance, can be seen in the area of leisure-recreation. Other problem areas in which the association is less strong include the patient's physical health, the patient as child caretaker, the family's relationship with relatives, family finances, the neurotic and overt behavior types of problems of children. Two illustrations of *moderate or extensive involvement with improvement* are given below.

1) Mrs. T. (two-parent) seemed to have more ego strength than many of the other demonstration patients. However, she fitted in well with the study population in terms of the need for consistent, aggressive, reaching-out efforts. As a frightened, isolated, and depressed young mother who feared that she could not function appropriately, she moved from literal flight from the demonstration worker to active participation, relating positively and with readiness to use relationship in building ego strength.

In regard to her role as a child caretaker (rated as moderate movement), she was given anticipatory guidance in relation to the development of her young son throughout the year. She was given a book and useful pamphlets on developmental tasks. She was

TABLE 21
Type of problem, Extent of involvement of demonstration worker, and movement

Type of Problem	Total with problem at beginning of year	Extent of involvement and movement							
		Minimal or none				Moderate or extensive			
		Total	Movement Unknown	None or deterioration	Improvement	Total	Movement unknown	None or deterioration	Improvement
Patient									
Health	25	15	4	8	3	10	2	3	5
Mental or emotional	35	6	0	2	4	29	1	13	15
As child caretaker	34	14	2	7	5	20	3 (a)	7	10
As homemaker	17	12	0	8	4	5	0	3	2
Employment	7	1	0	0	1	6	0	5	1
Father									
Health	18	12	5	6	1	6	0	5	1
Father-child relationship	18	17	2	14	1	1	0	0	1
Employment	12	9	1	4	4	3	0	2	1

Family								
Marital situation	7	1	4	2	18	2	10	6
Relationship with relatives	12	0	10	2	7	0	3	4
Leisure-recreation	15	0	11	4	11	0	3	8
Environmental								
Housing or neighborhood	22	1	13	8	5	0	3	2
Finances	19	3	11	5 (b)	13	0	7	6
Total families	35	35	35	35	35	35	35	35
Health	61	8	33	20	14	0	3	11
Neurotic traits	28	6	17	5	4	0	1	3
Behavior	27	3	20	4	8	0	3	5
School	33	6	21	6	1	0	0	0
Retardation	1	1	0	0	1	0	1	0
Sib relations	20	0	15	5	3	0	2	1
Peer relations	22	5	14	3	2	0	1	1
Total children	103	103	103	103	103	35	35	35

(a) Includes three cases showing a combination of improvement and deterioration within one family on separate items comprising the combined rating.
(b) Includes one case rated unknown for involvement.

encouraged to bring up concerns in order to develop a sense of the range of normalcy. She was given permission and helped to spend a part of her day in relating directly to her son. She was taught how to enjoy him, rather than ignoring him or being quick to pick up the negative. Patient was eager for this help and used it well with good carry-over. She moved during the year to develop a spontaneous, warm relationship with her son in which she could cuddle him and laugh with him.

In the area of *child health* (moderate movement) she was able to follow through on the major pediatric recommendations with a good deal of support and intervention from the demonstration worker. However, this required the worker's making the appointment for medical examination, driving mother and child to the hospital, and giving her money for the taxi fare home. She still had not completed basic immunizations by the end of the demonstration. Her pattern was to seek aid quickly in a crisis, but she had little grasp of the concept of preventive supervision.

The patient's difficulties in the leisure-recreation area were seen as a reflection of the mother's mental illness. The demonstration worker and patient worked in this area throughout the year. A great deal of emotional support was necessary before the mother could begin to move out of her isolation. Suggestions were made frequently by the worker as to how the mother could move out into the community. Whenever she made attempts to find interests with others, she received the worker's wholehearted support. Patient was able to move during the year from a desperate isolation, in which she literally had contact with no one outside her family, to being able to meet with other young people through her husband. In the end she could hold up her part of a social relationship, indicate her interest in wanting to see others again, and accept their invitations for future get-togethers.

2) Mrs. W. (two-parent) had been hospitalized on two occasions at _____ Hospital for a serious medical problem (subarachnoid hemorrhage from right internal carotid artery). After the second hospitalization and discharge she became quite depressed within a month, necessitating a psychiatric hospitalization (this study's key contact) at the same hospital. She was a patient there for about 3 weeks and was then transferred to _____ State Hospital where she remained for approximately 2 weeks, leaving against medical recommendation.

The patient was, however, able to continue through the demonstration year without the need for further psychiatric contact. In spite of a history of deprivation and rejection as a child, the physical and mental illnesses noted, and a low IQ, she progressed markedly in her ability to function during the year.

The patient's health improved considerably even though the situation was complicated by her depression (and, therefore, inability to look after herself as she should), pregnancy, and heavy smoking. The demonstration worker gave her considerable support and direct advice on follow-through in health supervision, prenatal care, and family planning. The worker coordinated her own efforts with the medical team at the _____ Hospital, and on doctors' recommendations obtained a homemaker before, furing, and after confinement. The extensive involvement in this one area had positive effects in other areas. These included mother's mental health, her adequacy as a child caretaker, and her adequacy as a homemaker.

COMMUNITY RESOURCES

Community agencies with which the demonstration and control families in the three studies had contact were grouped into seven basic types as follows: public assistance, children's agencies, family agencies, psychiatric services, correctional agencies, medical social services, and public health nursing. Psychiatric services included hospital or community after-care clinics, psychiatric outpatient clinics, mental health clinics, and child guidance clinics. Contacts with correctional agencies included those with court probation and parole officers, both adult and juvenile, and the state's services for juvenile delinquents.

Part of the task of the demonstration worker was to assist the family in making contact with appropriate social and health agencies in the community This was done through the process of referral, in accordance with the needs of the family. In addition, the demonstration worker undertook to coordinate her services and those provided by other agencies during the year through the media of case conferences and other types of contact. At the same time there were other agencies active with study families who were not contacted by the demonstration worker for specific reasons.

Agencies Active at Study Intake

The proportions of families in the three studies that were active with one or more of these seven agency types at the study intake, or that had been known to them in the past, were analyzed. One-parent families in all three studies had been or were currently known to public assistance agencies more frequently than to any other type of agency. In Study III this applied to 87.5% of the thirty-two one-parent families. Two-parent families were known to public assistance much less frequently, although this agency still represented one of the types that the families used the most often. Other agency types frequently utilized were family agencies for one-parent families in Studies II and III, children's agencies in all three studies, and parent groups except two-parent families in Study I, psychiatric agencies in all groups except control families in Study I because of the inclusion in that study of tuberculous patients, correctional and medical social services for one-parent families in Study III, and public health nursing agencies for all families except those in Study II.

One-parent families in Study III had contacts with community agencies, on the whole, more frequently than any other parent or study group and, in fact, seemed to have been relatively heavily dependent on all agency types. Contact with community psychiatric resources by two-parent families was, however, very frequent in Study II (29%), and in Study III the proportion (50%) exceeded that in one-parent families. The relatively small proportion of families with community psychiatric contacts in Study I was probably due to the controls which were chosen for tuberculosis rather than mental illness.

It was not clear why medical social services were not provided more frequently. Also the small number of contacts in Study II families with public health nursing services in suburban cities and towns was surprising in view of the relatively large proportions of families with such contact in each of the other two studies. The tuberculous condition of the controls in Study I required a more frequent utilization of public health nursing services than was true of mental patients, thus making Study I and Study II not comparable in this respect. It is possible, also, that greater reliance on a family physician in Study II may have provided some aspects of health supervision, such as immunizations, which were more likely to be provided through contacts with child health conferences and the public health nursing services in Study III. In any event, the failure of a nursing contact to be reported among even one of the twenty-two one-parent families in Study II must be considered unusual.

Over half of the 253 families (57%) were not known to any of the seven basic agency types. The proportion of two-parent white families who were not known to any basic type agency was relatively large for all studies and varied from 63 to 83%. The corresponding proportion for two-parent black families was considerably smaller (33%). Regardless of color, however, this proportion of families that had not used agencies was much greater for two-parent than for one-parent families in all studies. Only 8.5% of all families were active with agencies of two or more types. The majority of these were one-parent families. One-parent white families in Study III contributed especially to this group, one-third of the 24 families having been active with agencies of two or more types at the time of the study intake.

Agencies During Study Year

In Study II, the two small cities used as demonstration communities were selected partly because access to community resources might be more readily available than in the case of families in the towns used as control communities. It would therefore be expected that the demonstration families in both studies would have more contact during the year with community agencies than would the control families.

The number of families on whose behalf the demonstration workers in Study III developed contacts during the year with various types of community resources are shown in Table 22. The types of resources differ somewhat from the seven basic community agency types previously referred to in that contacts with hospitals concerning inpatients are included in the medical and psychiatric resources. The "all others" category comprises a number of formal and informal community resources that offered a limited or special type of social or health service but which were not considered basic welfare agencies. These included group work agencies of various kinds, Planned Parenthood services, Housing Authorities, Division of Employment, school departments, and the clergy. Private physicians and dentists were also included in this group because of their importance in the health maintenance of family members.

TABLE 22
Number of families concerning which
demonstration worker contacted at
least one agency of given type
(Study III)

Type of resource	Number of families concerning which demonstration worker contacted at least one agency of given type		
	Total	Two-parent	One-parent
Public assistance	18	5	13
Family agency	9	4	5
Child welfare	6	2	4
Psychiatric hospital (a) or clinic	28	14	14
Correctional	2	0	2
Medical hospital (a) or clinic	18	12	6
Public health nursing	4	3	1
All others	26	15	10
Total families	35	19	16

(a) Includes contacts regarding inpatients.

Except for the "all others" category the demonstration contacts took place most frequently with psychiatric and general hospitals and clinics, and with public assistance agencies. The frequent contact with psychiatric resources largely reflects the need for consultation about the patient's condition with the psychiatrist responsible for her treatment. The demonstration worker, surprisingly, made contact with the public health nursing service in only four instances, although eleven of the thirty-five families were active sometime during the study year with public health nursing services. Differences in the demonstration contacts according to one- or two-parent families are not remarkable except for public assistance agencies; their contact was made much more frequently for one-parent families (81%) than for two-parent families (26%) as would be expected because of the greater dependence of one-parent families on public assistance.

The proportions of thirty demonstration and forty-five control families with ill mothers in Study II, and of the thirty-five demonstration and thirty-five control families in Study III who were active with one or more of the seven basic types of agencies during the study year, are shown in Table 23. The criterion for judging "activity" differed somewhat by agency. Information on the activity of the family with an agency was obtained from the family by the research interviewer and from agency reports. Both sources were considered and checked against each other. Cases considered active at any given time were those in which there was evidence of recent contact and no indication from either source of a closing of such contact. The factor of recency of contact was considered in relation to agency type. For example, if the family noted that the public welfare worker or public health nurse usually visited about once every 6 months, this would be sufficient to establish that the case remained active even though there had been no contact for a period up to 6 months. On the other hand, if there was evidence that a patient, following a series of regular visits to a psychiatric clinic, had discontinued such visits for 3 months and had no further planned contacts, the case was considered closed.

TABLE 23
Families of ill mothers active with community agencies during year

Type of Agency (a) Study II (b) Study III	Total year Demonstration (N=30)(N=35)	Total year Control (N=45)(N=35)	At beginning and end of year Demonstration (N=30)(N=35)	At beginning and end of year Control (N=45)(N=35)	At beginning of year Demonstration (N=30)(N=35)	At beginning of year Control (N=45)(N=35)	At end of year Demonstration (N=30)(N=35)	At end of year Control (N=45)(N=35)	Within the year Demonstration (N=30)(N=35)	Within the year Control (N=45)(N=35)
Public assistance (a)	40%	16%	17%	2%	10%	0%	7%	2%	7%	11%
(b)	54%	43%	37%	29%	6%	6%	3%	3%	9%	6%
Children's (a)	7	11	3	2	0	0	0	4	3	4
(b)	11	17	0	6	3	0	3	6	6	6
Family (a)	37	11	17	0	3	4	13	4	17	2
(b)	20	20	0	9	0	3	9	3	11	6
Psychiatric (a)	67	67	9	11	3	13	20	20	27	31
(b)	69	57	9	2	3	3	26	26	31	17
Correctional (a)	7	9	0	2	0	2	7	4	0	0
(b)	14	6	6	0	3	3	3	0	3	3
Medical social service (a)	0	0	0	0	0	0	0	0	0	0
(b)	0	6	0	0	0	3	0	0	0	3
Public health nursing (a)	17	11	0	2	7	4	3	2	7	2
(b)	31	26	11	9	6	9	9	9	6	0

Contacts of demonstration and control families in both studies were more frequent during the year as a whole with community psychiatric resources than with any other agency type. In the majority of instances these contacts were made during the year and were not present at its beginning. Families continued to be at least active with medical social service and correctional agencies.

In comparing demonstration and control families who were known to agencies at any time during the year in Study II, it was found that the proportion of demonstration families exceeded that of the controls for public assistance and family agencies, with the other types showing very small or no differences. This difference for public assistance agencies was due mainly to the difference in the proportions of the two groups who were receiving assistance at the beginning of the year. On the other hand, the difference in the totals for family service agencies reflects mainly the relatively large proportion of demonstration, as opposed to control, families who became known through the efforts of the demonstration workers in referring families to these agencies during the study year. Counseling and/or homemaker services were offered by these family agencies to most of the demonstration families. It is of interest to note that the demonstration was successful in referring one family to a family service agency in the state of Virginia where the family had moved shortly before the end of the study year.

The fact that no difference appears in the proportion of demonstration and control families who were known to psychiatric agencies some time during the year resulted mainly from the difference between those active at study intake who discontinued contact during the year and those who did not. More demonstration than control families tended to retain their contacts. Thus, 17% of the demonstration and only 3% of the control families were in contact with such a service both at the beginning and end of the study year, while only 3% of the demonstration and 13% of the control families were known to at least one psychiatric service at the beginning of the year only. The proportion of demonstration families that ceased being active during the year was similar to that of controls for all agency types except for family service agencies, which discontinued a larger proportion of families active for an interval period only. Also, psychiatric services as noted above discontinued a somewhat smaller proportion of families that had been active at the beginning of the year.

The data for Study III showed that differences in the proportions of demonstration and control families active with various agency types some time during the year are less marked than in Study II. However, in Study III a larger proportion of demonstration than of control families became known to family service agencies during the year. These contacts by the demonstration families were mainly for the purpose of securing homemaker services. In contrast to Study II, however, psychiatric agencies discontinued contact with a somewhat larger proportion of demonstration than of control families, the difference reflecting more frequent short-term contacts by the demonstration group. No other differences relative to time of year were evident for other agency types.

One reason why no greater differences appeared between demonstration and control families in the use of community agencies in Study II was probably because both demonstration families and agencies saw the demonstration worker herself as a resource. This was true even though both the agencies and families knew that the demonstration was temporary; this fact undoubtedly resulted in a fewer number of demonstration families being serviced by community agencies.

The data in relation to use of agencies by the twenty-four families with ill fathers in Study II were examined separately. These twenty-four families were similar to those with ill mothers in that study, in that they were in contact with community psychiatric services during the year more frequently than with any other agency type. Six (60%) of the demonstration families and seven (50%) of the control families had such contacts, and in every instance they were initiated during the year. The families with ill fathers were also similar to those with ill mothers in that a larger proportion of the demonstration than of the control families were active with family agencies. This applied to four of the ten demonstration, as compared to none of the control families. Of the four demonstration families, one was active both at the beginning and end of the year, one at the beginning only, and two initiated contact during the year for interval periods only. While none of the twenty-four families with ill fathers was receiving public assistance at the point of hospitalization, seven families did initiate contacts with this agency during the year. There were no differences between demonstration and control families in this respect, and in all but two families these contacts had been discontinued by the year's end.

Agencies Discontinued

The circumstances associated with the discontinuance of contact by agencies were not systematically available in Study II. In Study III, however, the reason given most frequently by public assistance, children's, family, and psychiatric services for the closing of cases was the absence of further need for services. In view of the extensive social and health problems in these families as reported by the research interviewers and the demonstration staff, the frequency with which the absence of further need was given by agencies as a reason for closing was difficult to understand. However, agencies in closing cases appeared to be oriented to specific needs. Public assistance, e.g., would generally close its case if and when income maintenance was assumed by the family. In four of the six instances in which a family agency closed a case, the service of the agency had consisted primarily in providing a homemaker or another type of material assistance. When the acute need for this service disappeared, as when the patient returned from the hositpal, the service was withdrawn and the case closed. Children's agencies, too, seemed oriented primarily to meeting acute or emergency needs such as that for shelter when a parent was hospitalized. When immediate needs were met or the family presented difficulties in the use of service, there was a tendency on the part of agencies to discontinue treatment regardless of their awareness or lack of awareness of other underlying family problems.

Agencies' Awareness of Problems

In addition to assisting families in obtaining help from community resources, one of the aims of the demonstration was to emphasize to the agencies involved the importance of maintaining a preventive orientation in relation to a variety of problems concerning the health and welfare needs of children. It was expected, therefore, that agencies providing services to the demonstration families would, as a reflection of the total organization of the demonstration, be particularly cognizant of these needs. Three problem areas concerning finances, housing, and caretakers were considered to be especially significant for child-care. These areas were conceived of in broad terms, and any evidence of negatives or limitations from the research data were noted. Financial problems were noted when there was evidence of real difficulty due to limitations in the amount of income in relation to the size and material needs of the family. Income management problems related to inadequate budgeting procedures and the accumulation of excessive debts were also included. Housing limitations involved a wide variety of difficulties such as insufficient space for living or sleeping, dirty or filthy home conditions, neighborhood problems, and/or a realistic dissatisfaction for whatever reason with existing housing and a felt need to find new quarters. Limitations of caretakers, described in the preceding section, generally concerned (1) difficulties in relation to availability of time of the mother in Study III, or the mother and parent substitutes in Study II; (2) difficulties in their ability to cope with the physical (in Study III the physical and emotional) aspects of the caretaking process due to the health and adequacy components; and (3) their willingness to be a caretaker.

The number of families with limitations or difficulties in these areas at any time of the year was judged from the research data and the reports at the end of the year of one or more of the community agencies active with the family during the year. The agencies were simply requested to note any problems in the family perceived by them during the year, but were not specifically asked to list problems relevant to each of the three problem areas. It was therefore, not surprising that the proportion of families identified by one or more agencies as having difficulties in each of the three problem areas was smaller than that identified by the study. There was, however, no a priori reason to expect that the proportion of control families with difficulties identified by the agencies should be smaller than that of demonstration families. The data, however, indicate that this was, indeed, the case for all three areas, the difference approaching though not quite reaching significance ($X^2 = 3.3$, $P < .10$) in relation to income difficulties. These observations suggest, therefore, that these observed differences may have represented a heightened awareness of difficulties in these problem areas on the part of agency personnel participating in the demonstration. In nearly every instance in which agencies reported a problem, they also indicated that some attempt was made by them to be helpful.

In Study III the number of family and children's problems was expanded and classified into twenty areas relating to the patient, the father, the family as a whole, the environment, and the children. These areas included the three dealt with primarily in Study II. In order to maximize the comparability of data obtained from agency reports and from the study, comparisons were limited (1) to those families active with one or more agencies throughout the year for which agency reports were available at the beginning and at the end of the year; and

(2) to persistent problems, i.e., those reported at both times of the year by the study. With these limitations there were too few cases available for neamingful comparson of study data with those of children's, family service, medical social, and correctional agencies but comparisons were possible with public assistance, psychiatric, and public health nursing agencies. While the frequency with which any one problem reported both at the beginning and end of the year by the study was usually small, it was striking to find that those three types of agencies seemed relatively unaware of those problems relating to children. The same was true for marital and housing difficulties. For example, six families in which the public assistance agency was active at the beginning and end of the year had at least one child reported by the study to have neurotic traits. These children were most commonly described as "nervous," easily upset, poor sleepers, and poor eaters. Some problems were minimal in nature, while others were severe. In only one of these six instances was the agency aware of these difficulties at both times of the year, and in none of the other five instances did the agency become aware of them at any time during the year. A similar lack of awareness applied to psychiatric and public health nursing agencies in regard to their knowledge of children's neurotic traits. However, there was a slightly higher proportion of problems of demonstration than control families of which psychiatric and public health nursing agencies became aware during the study year.

It was not unusual for patients or families to have contact with more than one agency of a given type during the study year. This was particularly true of psychiatric and less frequently of medical services. The following is an illustration of a teen-age mother who had contact with three different psychiatric services.

O.L. (one-parent) was seen at the "A" Hospital emergency psychiatric service for initial contact. Within 2 weeks of this visit the demonstration worker became concerned regarding mother's bizarre talk. With patient's consent the demonstration worker escorted her back to the emergency psychiatric service for evaluation. Due to vague suicidal threats and obvious lack of control, the patient was referred to the "B" State Hospital where she was admitted. The demonstration worker continued contact with "B" State Hospital during mother's stay, which was short. The family did not agree with mother's hospitalization and encouraged her to leave. The mother was a difficult, unmanageable patient, and the "B" State Hospital did not support her staying. The demonstration worker tried to work with the hospital to enlist their interest in this most difficult teen-age mother, but without success.

Within a month after her return to the community, mother made another suicidal attempt. A friend summoned the police, and mother was taken to "C" Hospital Emergency Service and seen by a psychiatrist. She was kept in the hospital due to a gynecological infection, not for psychiatric reasons. The demonstration worker again tried very hard to work with this girl. The psychiatrist of this hospital conferred with the project staff concerning this case. It was his belief that the maternal grandparents constituted an exceptionally crucial factor in this situation and that, if they could not be reached, work with this mother would not be likely to yield results.

The mean number of resources contacted by the demonstration staff for the total of thirty-five families was six. This varies from 1.8 for eight of the families to 13.3 for three others. For ten of the thirty-five families, contacts were made with from nine to fourteen different community resources. Contacts with a community resource were frequently repeated and extended over periods of time during the study year.

Purpose of Demonstration Contacts with Agencies

Contacts with community resources were classified in relation to their purpose. The major purposes were information only, referral, and coodination of services. Coordination was defined to include case conferences, as well as any other kind of contact with a caseworker in the community agency concerning the management of a case. Contacts with psychiatric resources and public assistance agencies most frequently were for the purpose of coordination. Contacts of the demonstration worker for two or more different purposes, with two or more agencies of the same type, were made primarily with psychiatric resources. In nine of the twelve instances involved, coordination was also the purpose for contact with at least one agency. Contacts with family service agencies were most often for referral purposes, while those with a public health nursing service were mainly for information. On the other hand, contacts with medical hospitals or clinics involving only one resource were almost evenly divided among the three purposes. The following are some illustrations of contacts made by the demonstration worker for different purposes.

(1) Information only—public assistance

Mrs. N. (one-parent) was resistant and hostile to the demonstration worker at the time of her first visit. She requested that child be placed outside of the home. Due to the severity of the crisis and the number of agencies involved, the demonstration worker contacted all agencies before making demonstration plan in order to see how the demonstration could fit into the already ongoing complicated plan. Demonstration worker contacted mother's AFDC worker, who was very cooperative and helpful. This worker explained how the public assistance category would change from AFDC to general relief once the child was removed from the home, and what the financial implications of this change would be.

(2) Information only—medical

One child in the D. family (two-parent) had a hemophiliac condition which was being followed by the _____ Medical Center. Demonstration worker contacted the Center to learn of the present status of the child's health. The worker was informed that child was due for annual evaluation, and she helped mother to keep appointment for this evaluation. Later, the demonstration worker again contacted the Center to learn results of the visit. Results were normal, so that there was no need for further follow-up in this area.

(3) Referral—family service

The core problem for the D. family (two-parent) was seen as a need for marital counseling. The mother did not accept regular contact with the demonstration worker until the last 3 months of the project. At this point, due to time limitations, it seemed best to refer parents to an ongoing agency. The demonstration worker helped parents to face their needs, arrange a referral to the _____ Family Service, and supported the family through the intake procedure. Since the _____ Family Service was, however, unable to pick up the family for 3 months following intake, the demonstration worker continued with the case for this amount of time beyond the study year in order to provide continuity of service.

(4) Coordination—public assistance

Coordination in the G. case (one-parent) was consistently carried out with the AFDC worker throughout the year. The AFDC worker responded well and gave excellent service, in part perhaps because of the extensive support and interest that the demonstration worker showed.

With the demonstration worker's help, AFDC worker was able to see certain behavior (return of father) in the light of the mother's mental illness, rather than "going by the book" and therefore withholding assistance at critical points. With the demonstration worker's encouragement, AFDC worker brought services to the family (job training) and took part in community case conferences.

At the beginning, coordination with public assistance was facilitated by the demonstration worker's office being in the same building as that of the AFDC worker. This allowed for close contact. Both workers were then able to see mother (or both parents) when they visited the welfare office.

(5) Coordination—psychiatric

After the first month of contact, the demonstration worker contacted the _____ Hospital psychiatrist for clarification of Mrs. L.'s (two-parent) condition. The psychiatric history of the patient was discussed, and the psychiatrist helped the demonstration worker to define service areas in which to focus. He felt that the mother was not ready for employment, but requested that general support be given along with specific help with housing difficulties.

The demonstration worker had two further contacts with the psychiatrist during the year. In these contacts the worker and psychiatrist were able to check on the reality of mother's reporting in order to prevent her playing one professional person against the other, and to promote her understanding of reality.

Agency Contacts at End of Year

At the end of the study year, eleven demonstration families were formally referred to one of the basic types of community social or health agencies. One additional family was referred to two such agencies, making thirteen referrals in all for twelve families. Eight families were active during the year with a basic type agency (including, in one instance, a public housing authority) and continued active at the year's end, so that no new referral was necessary. The remaining fifteen demonstration families were not referred. Seven families refused referral when it was discussed with them. In two instances no referral was made due to an extended contact by the demonstration worker beyond the year's end. In the final six cases, referrals were not made because of individual family considerations, the most frequent of which was a family pattern of seeking help only on a crisis basis.

The thirteen referrals were distributed as follows: three to multiservice centers; three to general hospital outpatient departments, including one to the social service department; two each to family service agencies, mental health centers, and the public child welfare agency; and one to a division of legal medicine. It was expected and agreed to by the agencies at the time of referral that they would continue direct service in response to needs which had been demonstrated.

It was thought that there might be some degree of association between the choice of cases for referral and the initial degree of acceptance of the demonstration by the family. This was, in fact, not found to be the case. If anything, a somewhat larger proportion of those families who had initially shown a definite resistance or hostility to the demonstration were in the referred group, as compared to those who were not referred at the end of the year.

In the case of six of the thirteen referrals, the agency was still active with the family 8 to 15 months after the demonstration had closed. The agencies involved included three multiservice centers; two general hospital outpatient departments, including the social service department in one instance; and the public child welfare agency. In the later instance the agency had taken legal custody of a child. Regular contacts were made in only two of these six instances, the agencies involved being a multiservice center and a hospital outpatient department. In two others only a few contacts were reported, and at the time of inquiry the two multiservice centers concerned were about to close the cases. The frequency of contact with the family was not reported by the public child welfare agency in one of the remaining two instances, nor by a hospital social service department in the other.

One referral to the public child welfare agency had never been acted upon. In the remaining six of the thirteen referrals the agencies had closed the case at the time of the follow-up inquiry by this study. One family referred to a family service agency had been closed within 6 weeks of referral or after four interviews. The reason given for closing was failure by the client to follow through in maintaining contact with the agency. The other five cases were open for periods of from 4 to 6 months before closing. Contact had been regular in only two of these five instances. In one of these two cases the reason reported for closing by a division of legal medicine was that the worker had left the agency. In the second, the reason for closing was not reported, but it seemed likely that it was associated with the patient's hospitalization for a 30-day period of evaluation upon recommendation of a mental health center. In the other three instances contact between family and agency had been infrequent. In one case in which the referral had been to a mental health center, there had been only one interview in a 4-month period of activity. The reasons reported for closing in this case were failure of the patient to return and the decision not to reassign the case to a new worker after the death of the former one. In the second instance, involving a family service agency, the reason given for closing was again failure of the patient to follow through, and in the third instance the patient discontinued contact with a hospital psychiatric outpatient department because she felt it was not helpful.

The agencies provided an estimate of the problems for seven of the thirteen referrals. Some of the main problems which they saw included marital conflict, or need of marital counseling, psychiatric illness, including a severe character disorder, a mother's need to divorce herself emotionally from her children in order to allow them to lead their own lives, and retardation of a child. The agency's evaluation agreed generally with that of the demonstration in five of the seven instances.

The six agencies which had closed their cases at the time of inquiry were asked about the occurence of crises in families referred to them during the time in which they had been active. In only four instances was a definitive reply given. Noted was a suicidal attempt, a pregnancy and mental hospitalization in the case of a divorced woman, a "constant crisis," and "no outstanding crisis." In the other two instances the agency worker stated that she did not know.

In the twelve instances in which the agencies had had contact with the family, they reported success in treatment in two cases, partial or limited degree of success in three, no success in five instances, unknown in one instance, and in the final case data was not available. Prognosis was considered good in only two instances, although in another case it was considered good for the children, and in a third the family was described as making progress. In four instances prognosis was described as poor, guarded, or difficult. In the remaining instances prognosis was unknown or information was not available.

Community agencies active with Study III families during the study year were asked to identify difficulties which they encountered in providing services. The replies were surprising in that public assistance, family service, child welfare, psychiatric, and public health nursing agencies reported no difficulties for one-half or more of the families known to them. Psychiatric agencies were active with more families than any other agency type and were the only type that permitted the categorization of difficulties for any appreciable number of families. Among forty-four patients known to psychiatric agencies, twenty-three were reported as offering no difficulties, eleven as not keeping appointments or being otherwise uncooperative, two as having difficulty in accepting help or forming relationships, two as showing other types of difficulties, and data were not available for the remaining seven patients.

There appeared to be several factors associated with the agencies' failure to report more fully on difficulties encountered in working with these families. Perhaps the most general one was the failure of agencies to become involved in many of the family problems even though they were aware of them. In some instances this was the result of a realistic decision on the agencies' part. For example, in at least two instances the failure of a family agency to make note of any difficulties seemed to be associated with the fact that, after brief contact, referrals were made to a psychiatric agency. In another instance a public health nursing service, aware that the family had multiple social and health problems for which help was being provided through other agencies, noted only in relation to their own limited role that the patient was a "good clinic mother."

It seems likely, however, that agencies might have reported more difficulties had they seen their role as one requiring a more thorough involvment with a range of family and children's problems. Such a role might well have been characterized by a more aggressive referral and follow-up policy, coordinated treatment in the case of families being seen by more than one agency, and reduced caseloads. For example, a public assistance worker reported that her client had difficulty budgeting within her AFDC allowance but, due to a heavy caseload, the worker did not have time to help her with this. The worker went on to note that the children had many health problems, but that the family had always hesitated to call doctors, go to hospitals, or buy drugs because of lack of money In another instance in which no difficulties in rendering services were reported, the worker expressed the opinion that the family would make progress only after their health problems were put in check. There was, however, no information to indicate that this worker was helpful to the family in accomplishing this goal. In still another instance, the welfare worker noted that "the family required motivation for the use of all services available."

The reluctance of families to turn to social or health agencies, whether because of financial difficulties or other reasons, was a not uncommon phenomenon of which agencies in the field were aware. In describing a family, one public assistance worker reported: "It is my belief that this family will use services that are available only when and if they understand what they will gain. They have complained that they do not like so many people concerned about them. If they can be convinced that all contacts are made for their benefit, I am sure they will cooperate." Another family on public assistance was described as poorly motivated toward the use of public medical services and preferred to use private services which were responsible for a major portion of their indebtedness.

In some instances families were known to be in treatment with a second agency, and the failure to report difficulties seemed to be associated with a limitation, justified or not, in the assumed role of the primary agency. A public health nursing service reported tha a mother discontinued giving her 1-year-old, retarded child with PKU a diet that had been medically prescribed because it was "too much bother." Although the mother was obviously neglecting this child and her other children, there were no indications in the nursing notes of difficulties in providing services to this family or of action taken by the nursing agency. A different type of situation was reported by a public assistance worker who noted that her client "has difficulty functioning as a homemaker, as she is emotionally upset attempting to keep numerous medical, dental, and psychiatric appointments at the _____ Hospital." Again, there was no indication that the worker became involved in this problem.

On the whole, therefore, it would appear that agencies might have reported more difficulties if they had a more complete understanding of the situation in the families and if they had interpreted their roles more broadly. However, in spite of limitations in agency roles, the great majority of the demonstration and control patients for whom information was available reported that agencies had been very helpful to them and their families.

Effectiveness of Agencies' Services

Each agency with which the demonstration staff had had contact during the year was rated in relation to its effectiveness from the point of view of meeting the needs of the family. Effectiveness of service was judged in relation to four factors: agency policy, agency practice, motivation of family, and continuity of the services provided. Ratings of the adequacy of medical and psychiatric practice in hospitals or clinics were meant to reflect such factors as interest shown in the medical or psychiatric problems of the patient or family, follow-up on pediatric recommendations of the project pediatrician, cooperation with the family and demonstration, and organization of services, rather than actual medical competence of individual physicians. The number of families who received ineffective services is given in Table 24. These services are classified by type of resource and factors associated with ineffectiveness. It can be seen that services judged to be ineffective were most frequently due to inadequate practice on the part of the practitioner and to lack of motivation on the families' part, regardless of the type of resource. The following examples provide illustrations of the four factors associated with ineffective service.

(1) Inadequate policy—psychiatric service

After the initial emergency contact, Mrs. U. (two-parent) was referred to the _____ Psychiatric Outpatient Department. After one interview by a social worker, the OPD reported that patient was

TABLE 24
Number of families receiving ineffective services by types of
community resources and factors associated with ineffectiveness

Type of resource	Total families represented by contacts (a)	Total with ineffective services (b)	Associated factors				
			Inadequate policy	Inadequate practice	Family "not motivated"	Service not continuous	Unknown
Public assistance	18	9 (c)	3	6	2	0	1
Family agency	9	6 (c)	0	5	5	0	1
Child welfare	6	3	1	3	2	0	0
Psychiatric hospital or clinic	28	19	11	15	16	9	0
Correctional	2	2	0	2	1	0	0
Medical hospital or clinic	18	9	2	6	6	1	2
Public health nursing	4	0	0	0	0	0	0
Total families	35	35	35	35	35	35	35

(a) Between demonstration staff and community resources.
(b) Rows do not add since more than one factor may be involved for each family.
(c) Does not include one case in which the raters were unable to judge adequacy of services provided.

untreatable. This decision appears to have been influenced also by the opinion of a second social worker in the OPD who had known the patient as a child, and who felt that she could not be helped. After a brief informal conversation between the social worker and the demonstration worker, the case was closed at the hospital OPD.

Factors possibly relating to agency policy which seem to have been associated with the limitations of service to this very needy family include (1) a judgment of untreatability made after only one interview by a social worker, after a referral by a psychiatrist in the emergency service who had apparently felt that further psychiatric help was indicated; and (2) the failure of the hospital staff to accept responsibility for working out alternative arrangements, together with the demonstration, for help for this patient and/or supervision of the children.

(2) Agency policy—psychiatric service

Mrs. T. (two-parent) originally had contact with the _____ Hospital Psychiatric Outpatient Department, but was transferred to another hospital for equivalent services during the course of the year. The transfer seemed to have been made for no other reason than that the psychiatrist involved found the work with this client too difficult. This mother needed a reaching-out type service including home visiting, which was not provided. The service offered by both hospitals in this case was judged to be poor. The father was never included in any way, although there were indications that he should have been. It was left to the demonstration worker to fill gaps in service for which the hospital clearly had an obligation.

While it was difficult to separate policy and practice in this instance, policy was rated as other than adequate in view of (1) an unnecessary transfer of the case from one hospital to another, which seemed to have implications for policy; and (2) the raters' understanding that neither hospital provided home visiting services.

(3) Agency policy—public assistance

Mrs. W. (two-parent) applied for AFDC in Town A in August, 1965. She was told to wait for an investigation. During September she moved to Town B before being put on the Town A welfare rolls. This necessitated her going through the whole routine again with the Town B welfare office. No one came to this woman's rescue with emergency help. Town A felt no responsibility for mother as she had never received her first check from then, even though in a move from one town to another all towns have the responsibility to carry a mother for 30 days while the new town sets up the new applications. Town B felt no responsibility for the emergency, saying that Town A was supposed to carry mother for 30 days. As a result of the inability of the welfare system to meet the client's needs on a crisis basis, the family was kept waiting for financial assistance, including rent payments, for 2 months. [As of July, 1968, this problem would not have existed because of the assumption by the State of the responsibility for all needy families.]

(4) Inadequate practice—child welfare

The V. children (two-parent) were referred by the demonstration in January, 1966, to the public child welfare agency for immediate temporary shelter on an emergency basis. Circumstances included admission of the patient, who was pregnant, to hospital for hepatitis; a history of child-battering by the father, in whose care the patient did not wish to leave the children; and a maternal great-grandmother, who was available for emergency child-care, but who drank excessively and had dropped the baby in the past. Children were placed temporarily in her care pending action by the child welfare agency.

Within the month mother delivered a stillborn child and was discharged home from the hospital. Placement of the children had still not been effected and continued to be requested due to the nature of the hepatitis convalescence. Both the principal supervisor and intake supervisor were contacted by the demonstration worker to no avail. Six weeks later the mother abandoned her family for 4 days, stating upon her return that she had consciously done this in order to pressure the children's agency to remove her children. This was relayed to the intake supervisor.

One month prior to termination of the demonstration, as a result of great pressure brought to bear by the demonstration worker, the children's agency reported that they had visited the home three times without finding the mother in, a problem which the demonstration worker had only infrequently found during her year-long visits. At the termination of the demonstration year in May, 5 months after the initial contact, the children's agency had still taken no action. This was true even though the demonstration worker had complained of possible battering in the interim.

(5) Inadequate practice—psychiatric service

Mrs. D. (two-parent) informed the demonstration worker that, following her emergency visit to the hospital, she had been referred to the psychiatric outpatient department. She was seen for diagnostic purposes, at which time a panel of doctors was in attendance. She was given to understand that she was on the waiting list, and was told by a doctor that someone would visit the home to discuss marital problems with her and her husband.

The demonstration worker visited the psychiatric outpatient department twice in the second month after patient's initial contact, and once again 2 months later. At first she was told that the patient was on a waiting list, but no one seemed able to verify this. When the demonstration worker indicated her interest in having the outpatient department follow through with service to the patient, she was told that the patient would have to wait several months due to turnover of resident staff. By the 4-month period, the case seemed clearly "lost," as no one knew of the patient.

(6) Inadequat practice—public assistance

Mrs. D. (one-parent) was a masochistic woman, well able to "arrange" difficulties in her relationships with others. The public assistance worker seemed unaware of the severe pathology in this family, was consistently hostile and unnecessarily withholding in her relationships with the patient. She handled the three disturbed boys in the family by threatening them if they did not cooperate.

In this situation difficulties easily arose in the relationship between the welfare worker and the family. For example, the mother had requested a new stove for some time. Due to depression and masochism she was unable to follow regular procedure, i.e., obtain an estimate and have the welfare office authorize it. Rather than finding a way past the mother's obstruction, the public assistance worker played into it. Although the demonstration worker spent considerable time in consultation with the public assistance worker during the year, no progress was made in helping her to a better understanding of this family.

(7) Family not motivated—family service

Mrs. T. (two-parent) was quite threatened and fearful in her contacts with social agencies, possibly due to extensive contact which her family had with them during her own childhood. However, prior to her confinement the hospital requested that homemaker help be provided because of her poor health. This was arranged following a number of contacts by the demonstration worker with both the family service agency and the hospital.

The patient was able to accept this help until she returned home with the baby. She had been advised to retain homemaker assistance following her return home and arrangements had been made for this. However, she refused help within the first week after coming home. Later she became quite sick, possibly due to exhaustion in caring for the new baby.

(8) Services not continuous—psychiatric service

At the point of initial contact with the emergency service, Mrs. M. (two-parent) was transferred to the _____ State Hospital. Less than a month later she was returned home, but without provision for follow-up care. On the day when the demonstration worker made her inital home visit, the patient said that she felt depressed and was going to phone the hospital social worker. The hospital was cooperative in sharing information with the demonstration worker. However, they showed no initiative in follow-up with the patient even when told of her depression.

The patient was hospitalized two more times during the year following visits to the same emergency service from which she had been hospitalized the first time. The second time she was taken to a different state hospital. The third time she was kept at the general hospital following her emergency visit, probably due to her physical condition as a result of a suicidal attempt. This case illustrates not only the lack of continuity of psychiatric service from any one source, but also the lack of coordination between various psychiatric facilities and the duplication in the use of hospital services.

Thus, in general, there was inadequate coordination of community services. Also agencies closed their cases soon after the families were referred to them and before very much could be accomplished. With the seriousness of the problems involved, a longer and more continuous contact with these multi-problem families was necessary if any lasting results were to be obtained.

8

Impressions of the Study Staff

The research interviewers, demonstration social workers, and the pediatrician in Study III were all requested to formulate their impressions of the study population, their own experiences, including problems encountered in their work, and their own thinking concerning the further development of methods for carrying forward the objectives of the study. The purpose of this chapter is simply to present the views of the staff. Although each of the two research interviewers and four of the five demonstration workers presented separate reports, these were integrated within each of these two staff groups for purposes of presentation.

THE RESEARCH INTERVIEWERS

The two research interviewers in Study III faced a particularly difficult task. They were required to find and make the initial contact with the patient, who was often in a disturbed state following the visit to the emergency service, complete the initial interview, explain the study, and secure the family's agreement to the pediatric examinations and, in the demonstration families, to the visit of the demonstration social worker. Both interviewers were qualified social workers. Both had their master's degree in social work, and each had a number of years of experience in casework. One of the two interviewers had been employed as an interviewer in Study II, and was able to attest to differences in the interviewing experiences between the two studies. Both interviewers were painstaking and thorough in their efforts to locate families, secure the needed information, and motivate the family to participate in the study. The fact that so many of the families eligible for the study were found and agreed to participate is in no small measure due to their efforts.

Difficulties in Locating Patients

The first research interviews in the home with patients visiting the emergency service were made without prior announcement. It was felt that this policy would minimize the delay in making the first contact with the study families, and would lessen the chances that the family might decide against participation if announcement was first made by telephone or letter. In point of fact it soon turned out that many families did not have telephones and that finding or locating the family presented a real problem. The reasons for this varied, and some of the difficulties in locating patients in the deprived urban areas were described by one of the interviewers:

Firstly, addresses hurridly taken by the attending physician in the emergency wards in both hospitals used were occasionally erroneous. Either no such address existed, or the patient did not live at the address given. Secondly, a large proportion of the houses we visited were in the poorer sections of the city. There were no doorbells, no name plates on the doors, and it was frequently impossible to determine whether or not a patient actually lived at a given address. Usually knocking on a neighbor's door was the only way that we could ascertain whether or not a patient actually lived there. When, as so frequently happened, there was no one at home on any of the floors of the house, this meant another visit on another day just to determine this. We found a great mobility among our patient load. Families frequently moved from one address to another, leaving no forwarding address with neighbors or with the local post office. Locating such patients became a job of detection and often we were unsuccessful.

As the weather grew warmer, our chances of finding a patient at home anytime during the day grew even slimmer. The research area bounds the city beaches and the patients apparently flocked to the beaches in the warm weather. For example, on one day in August four patients were not in and only one, who was hospitalized at _____ Hospital, was available to be seen. Since this patient refused to participate in the research project, this was a wasted day. Although it seemed likely that the beaches accounted for the patients' whereabouts in the summertime, as the weather grew colder we were also unable to locate patients, and we did not understand where the patients went. Even when the patient was hospitalized it was not always possible to complete an initial interview in one visit, due to the patient's condition or other reasons.

When a mother was hospitalized, the research interviewers were requested to visit the caretaker of the children. This sometimes involved complications in the community as well as with the patient in the hospital. This is seen in the following example cited by one of the interviewers:

Mrs. B., an attractive, intelligent mother of five children, was taken to the emergency ward of the _____ Hospital by police after trying to board a plane to California with the five children, claiming she was on her way to marry a nationally known singer. She was transferred to _____ Hospital, at which point I tried to visit the patient at this hospital, but was informed by the nurse that she was still too disoriented to converse rationally with anyone. She suggested I call again in a week. Although we knew patient's mother was caring for her children, we were uncertain where the children were. Accordingly, I began by visiting the patient's home. As I found no one home, I decided that the children were probably in another town with their grandmother. A trip to this town in the late afternoon proved futile as I was unable to locate the address.

The following day I tried the address again, and this time I actually located the grandmother's home. Again there was no answer to my ring, but an upstairs neighbor who had seen me approach came down to tell me that the grandmother had been home for 2 days with the children to get some clean clothes, and had departed again for the patient's home where she intended to stay with the children. Later that afternoon I went back to the patient's apartment, but again found no one home. Four days later while at the hospital on another visit, I inquired about the patient. Although better oriented, she was still mute and still unable to answer questions. The nurses stated spontaneously that Mrs. B. was a very nice girl and that her mother came every afternoon to see her. This explained the mother's absences from the apartment. Under these circumstances, I planned my next visit to patient's apartment for a morning and this time found patient's mother at home. Four days later I returned to the hospital and this time was actually able to see the patient. However, as the interview progressed it was obvious that she was still hallucinating, and I terminated the interview while making arrangements to return again. After seven visits I was finally able to complete the initial interview.

One other extreme example of the mobility of these patients and the difficulty in locating them is given below:

The original address of the D. family in the hospital record proved to be an abandoned building. I went up and down in front of it, because sometimes part of a seemingly abandoned building is inhabited. However, there weren't any signs of life and the windows were boarded up. When I reported this to the case finder, she got in touch with _____ Hospital and got a new address for the D. family. The block began typically with a bar and then some other businesses. This block, too, seemed partially abandoned and ended in a vacant lot. It was on the edge of a redevelopment area, and I thought the number might be on the other side of the torn up area. I passed a church left standing in the middle of the rubble, and continued on until I came to an industrial area. Here the numbers were higher than the one that the hospital had given as the D.'s address. Obviously, the D.'s had at one time lived in a building which had been torn down.

When I reported this to the case finder, she again got in touch with the hospital and was given a third address. I succeeded in interviewing Mrs. D. at this last address on the first try, and found that they had lived at the other addresses previously. They were now temporarily staying with friends.

The study pediatrician and I stopped at this address some time later to arrange a pediatric visit and found the D.'s had moved again. The D.'s friends weren't sure where they were now, but said that Mr. D. stopped in off and on and they would take down the new address and I could come back and get it. I did this later, and the D.'s friends were able to provide a specific address this time. I did not find Mrs. D. but was told by a pleasant and seemingly unsuspicious woman that a lady answering her description was believed to have moved out about 2 weeks ago, but her address was unknown. This happened to be next door to the office of a neighborhood organization and I thought it was possible that the D.'s had been there for some reason. I went in and talked to the young woman in charge, who looked through the files but could find no record of contact with the D.'s. She could think of no way of tracing the D.'s except through the post office. I went to the one that she said was nearest, found no delivery of mail was done from this office, and the next day I visited the proper office. No forwarding address had been left by Mrs. D. The post office volunteered to ask the carrier to make inquiries in the building where she was last believed to have lived, but they were very doubtful of any results. The postal clerk spoke of how people moved around not leaving addresses, and that this was something that went on all the time in this area. When I checked back later, they had not been able to find the D.'s.

I did find them more or less by accident. I was in the neighborhood seeing another patient and decided to go to the hospital to look up records that might give an address for the D.'s. In the course of finding what proved to be a valid address, I was sent to five different offices in the hospital. It was only because Mr. D. had been a surgical patient in the clinic that very morning that I got the new address. I stopped and told the post office about this, and the clerk gave me a change of address card to give Mrs. D. I went to the new address, but found no one home.

A day or two later, I visited again and Mrs. D. saw me before I saw her. She was leaning out the window, greeted me in a very friendly way, and came down at once to open the door. It was evident that Mrs. D. had no idea of the procedure of leaving forwarding addresses.

I had arranged with Mrs. D. about a pediatric appointment, but when the study pediatrician went to see the children the family had moved again, and their whereabouts were unknown. A letter with a return receipt requested was sent to Mrs. D., but the family wasn't found. I hadn't felt too confident that she would follow through on leaving her forwarding address, and my lack of confidence was justified. Some time later while in the neighborhood for other reasons, I talked with the principal of the school that the D. children would have attended, had they not made this last move. She had never heard of the children but was most cooperative in making suggestions. She suggested that a local realty company might know something about this family. I went to this company immediately and learned that the D.'s had not rented any apartment through them, but oddly enough the realty owner at once recognized the family from my description.

I again checked with the hospital sometime later but officials there did not have any new addresses. As a last resort, I was able to have a check made by several school attendance officers through the cooperation of the city school committee. After lengthy inquiry, these officers also were unable to locate the family, which finally had to be dropped from the study.

Attitude of the Patient to the Interview

The attitude of the patients toward the research interview and the study varied greatly. Outright refusals of the initial interview, however, were rare. One of the reasons for this appeared to be that patients received the interviewer as a representative of the hospital in which they had so recently been served. The nature of their relationship with the hospital, however, as determined by their previous experience with it appeared to affect their attitude to the Study. If their previous experiences with the institution had been positive, they were likely to be receptive to the interviewer. Many patients, however, had a tenuous relationship with the hospital. Some had no intention of going back and were quite reluctant to participate in the Study. Most of the patients, nevertheless, accepted the interviewer, perhaps because they did not know how to avoid it. It was recognized, too, that some patients might have felt ashamed of events leading up to their visit to the emergency service and of having seen a psychiatrist. They were, perhaps understandably, not eager to discuss this. In contrast, a number of other patients were noticeably anxious to talk. This was illustrated in the following account by one of the interviewers:

Mrs. B. denied the suicide attempt by saying that she had taken too many headache pills, and really couldn't remember anything about the entire episode. Mrs. T. was ashamed of her suicide attempt, as was Mrs. N., and they were most reticent to discuss it. In many cases such patients as these had no intention of returning to the hospital, and could see no relationship between the interviewer and their visit to the hospital. Such patients participated most reluctantly in the research interview, and many of them would have refused had they known how to do so gracefully. Some patients who were reluctant answered questions put to them, but volunteered very little information and much of their material was guarded and evasive.

On the other hand, many patients were full of their personal problems and were most anxious to talk to anyone who would listen. Among such patients was Mrs. T., isolated and lonely, who welcomed the opportunity to talk about herself with the worker, and wanted to claim the research interviewer as her social worker. Mrs. H., a much younger woman but also isolated from the world, looked on the 4-month interview as a social event by serving coffee and cookies and enjoying the opportunity to discuss herself and her problems. Mrs. D., also a compulsive talker, enjoyed ventilating her many physical symptoms. She accepted the worker easily because she had been going to the _____ Hospital for many years and felt completely at home there. Later, when it turned out that this patient did not have a psychiatric diagnosis but was actually suffering from a bleeding ulcer from which she nearly died, her attitude toward the hospital was completely negative and she used the 4-month interview to ventilate these negative feelings. Mrs. C. was very hostile to the hospital, but this did not prevent her accepting the research interview readily. Mrs. E. was also a compulsive talker and she, too, talked about herself to anyone. This woman welcomed the opportunity to complain about what she considered wretched treatment at the hospital.

Those who accepted the interview in a positive way varied considerably in their motivation and approach. Mrs. G., for example, seemed to be really asking for help with her own problems of personal and family adjustment. To be sure, she was glad to talk, but was not as compulsive as the patients previously mentioned. Both Mrs. I. and Mrs. P. were reserved in manner, did not usually share their troubles with others, and had considerable strength. Both accepted the idea of participating in the study and were even more sharing in the second interview. In contrast, Mrs. N. and Mrs. Q. did not need to talk, but were ready to discuss the emergency service experience. Mrs. M. and Mrs. R. both appeared willing, but not eager. However, these two mothers were friendly, moderately talkative women who welcomed a break in their routine.

Patients varied also in relation to the personal meaning which the interview had for them and the ways in which they used it. This was shown in the following account:

For Mrs. N., who could not tolerate the presence of a delinquent son in the home, the interview was a welcomed opportunity to ventilate her feelings. Mrs. P., who had recently told her daughter that she was illegitimate, was so upset by the experience that she had to be taken to the emergency ward a the city hospital. She was anxious to tell her side of the story, thereby relieving her guilt. By the 4-month interview this situation had worked out well. This time the patient was less accepting of my visit.

Mrs. T., who was most reluctant to participate in the initial interview, had the opposite experience at 4 months. Having decided to remain with her husband, she was experiencing many problems about which she was anxious to talk.

In general, patients tended to be more reluctant to participate in the research interview as the crisis in their lives receded. As they were more able to cope with their problems, they were less interested in talking with the research interviewer. For instance, Mrs. E., a young unmarried mother of two small children was extremely fearful that I would take the children away. Mrs. G., whose 3-year-old son had been seriously hurt in an accident, was hospitalized at the time of the initial interview. She suspected that her adequacy as a parent was being questioned, and was therefore reluctant to talk even though she consented to an interview.

There was no consistent relationship between the attitude of the patient in the first interview and that at the 4-month and year periods. Some who had been very accepting of the initial interview were hostile at the later ones, while the reverse was also true. Others were uniformly hostile or accepting. It was felt, however, that patients who had had considerable contact with the social workers in the past were able to talk more clearly with the interviewers than those who had not, while those who had difficulty relating were also poor respondents. Those who had not gone to the emergency service of their own free will tended, understandably, to be less accepting of the interview. One interviewer, in addition, noted her impression that patients more readily accepting the interview tended to be those most able to express concern about their children and the possible effect of their own problems on their children.

THE DEMONSTRATION STAFF

The demonstration social workers were required to visit the patient and members of the family as soon as possible after the research interview had been obtained in order to offer social services to meet critical needs associated with the patient's visit to the emergency service. Beyond providing the immediate or crisis services to families, however, the following longer term goals were formulated:

(1) To identify the social, psychological, health, and school problems of the group of children whose mothers were mentally ill;

(2) To involve community agencies in helping to meet the problems of children and of parents. This was to be accomplished through helping families to use community services, as well as through coordination of such services and community planning;

(3) To find new patterns of service for meeting the above needs, and to help in improving or developing facilities for such service.

The demonstration staff included a maximum of three professional social caseworkers at any one time during the study year. Due to staff turnover, however, five workers in all worked on the demonstration. All five were caseworkers with the master's degree in social work, while one had her doctorate, and another had completed a third year in casework at a school of social work. Their years of experience varied in number from 4 to 18, with three of the five workers having also had previous supervisory or administrative experience. All were committed to the purposes of the Study. They consistently made attempts to reach out to the families for whom they were responsible and were persistent in their efforts to provide needed services.

After the first 4 months of work with the families the demonstration staff reviewed their experiences and recorded their impressions. The strongest impression of the staff was that of the resistance of the families and the difficulty in engaging the mothers in a casework relationship. In contrast to Study II in which the first contact of the demonstration workers was with the patient's relatives, the demonstration workers in Study III found themselves immediately involved with the patients symptomatology. The mental illness of the parents, the extremely poor living conditions, and the multiplicity of problems proved distressing to the demonstration workers.

In about one-fourth of the families the demonstration seemed to represent to the mother the threat of taking the children away from her. This was either implied or said directly by the mother. The staff was also impressed by an immature quality in these mothers unrelated to chronological age. Patients seemed more like daughters than mothers, or more like adolescents than mature women able to mother their children. Many of the patients spoke quite openly of the loss of their own mothers as a background of their current difficulties.

Although more than half the families had prior agency contacts, the demonstration workers were impressed with the fact that at the point of crisis the hospital seemed to be the only community institution to which they turned. They also noted that some families which had extensive contacts with social agencies had learned to be very manipulative, and that this was early reflected in the family's relationships with them as well.

Because of the extent of the mothers' needs the demonstration workers found themselves hampered in their attempts to provide direct services for children. However, the pediatric examinations did provide one opportunity for focusing upon the children's health needs. Nevertheless, mothers were frequently not ready to follow through on the pediatric recommendations. This raised an important methodological question, i.e., whether to arrange directly for children to receive the necessary medical services or whether to wait and support the mother in finding a way to fulfill this responsibility, herself, as a parent.

Although the original demonstration plan called for a caseload of twenty families with mentally ill mothers, the demonstration workers felt that this was too large to permit full and continuous engagement with family members and with community resources. In view of this, the plan was revised so that the demonstration caseload did not exceed fifteen families. The demonstration workers also recognized the need for continuing psychiatric consultation. This was met in part by the hospital psychiatric staffs. In addition, a senior psychiatrist on the staff of one of the hospitals was designated as a liaison member by the department of psychiatry.

The demonstration workers reported that one of the most significant ways of providing help in this beginning period was in supporting the mother while she waited for a return appointment to the outpatient department and in helping her decide to keep this appointment. Other help included homemaker service, day care and day camp services, and, in some instances, assistance with clinic visits for children. A great many contacts with a variety of community agencies were also made.

Throughout the study year one of the greatest problems facing the demonstration workers was the mental state of the mother. Workers felt that they were hampered in all their efforts by the mother's mental instability and great emotional needs. Until the mother responded to psychiatric treatment, the demonstration workers felt that efforts to help in other areas (e.g., employment, family planning, provision of children's services) would not be successful.

One demonstration worker at the end of the study described her mothers as a "chronic group." They were seen as women who were deprived and rejected by their own mothers and for whom this mother-daughter relationship remained as a major problem in adult life. Two demonstration workers reported that their families were socially isolated, although the third failed to see isolation as a problem in view of the activity of extended families and informal neighborhood groups. Some mothers who were not hospitalized during the year were believed by the demonstration workers to have needed hospitalization. Regardless of whether hospitalization was indicated, however, it was felt that more consistent and readily accessible psychiatric services should be available.

In addition to the pressing need for psychiatric services, many comments were made by the demonstration workers concerning the lack of other community services available to these families. The two hospitals themselves from which patients had been drawn were felt not to be meeting the needs of these mothers. Hospitals were described as having no consistent follow-up plan. There was little communication and coordination among various clinics. One demonstration worker noted that this was to be regretted because these patients wanted the hospital to care. In fact, when the demonstration workers introduced themselves initially as representing the hospital, it gave the mothers hope that the hospital was now ready to provide the needed services. One worker suggested that one of the reasons that these families had failed to obtain needed services was that professional persons had turned away from them in self-defense.

In part because of the absence of follow-up service from the hospital, it was suggested that the use of agencies located in the neighborhood or physically close to the family might be more successful than attempted referral to hospitals. An example was given of families who lived in the area served by one of the mental health clinics with which the project was associated. These families were able to accept a referral to the clinic much more easily than to the outpatient department of a hospital or to a social agency in an "intown" location.

School services were felt to need strengthening, as did also programs for housing, employment, and neighborhood planning. The need for day-care services was found to be particularly acute. One shocking example of lack of services was that of a state program for delinquent youth that returned home a very disturbed boy who was a definite threat to himself, other children in the family, and to the community.

The demonstration workers evaluated their own work at the close of the study year. The original design of the Study had called for each of the three demonstration social workers to have an office in one of the participating agencies in different areas of the city, a public welfare office, a neighborhood center, or a mental health center. As the demonstration developed, however, it became increasingly impractical to use these offices, and their physical identification with these agencies was discontinued. This result may have been associated with the fact that the primary identification of the demonstration workers was with the Study rather than with the several agencies. However, the demonstration workers felt that the demonstration would have been more successful and easier for clients to accept if it had operated as an integral part of an established neighborhood agency. One of the advantages of such an arrangement would have been the probable avoidance of gaps in service, such as unfortunately occurred due to staff turnover during the demonstration. Also the clients would have had confidence that someone would have filled in when needed, especially in crisis situations.

The workers generally felt that 1 year was too short a time in which to effect change in a study population characterized by illness, economic deprivation, and long-standing multiple social problems. One worker offered as evidence for this the results obtained when she extended her services for several months after the close of the demonstration year. Although a "tapering off" period of several months in the study was provided, it was felt that the year of the demonstration left some families without support at a time when it was still needed and could have been profitably utilized. Unfortunately, some of these families were not ready for a referral to a community agency when contact with the project had to be finally terminated. In the absence of a definite problem or crisis at the termination point, referral tended to be resisted both by the families and the agencies. Even when the family was ready to accept a referral, however, the referral process was frequently time-consuming and hampered by red tape or restrictive agency policies.

There was question as to the advisability of a caseload consisting entirely of multiproblem and mentally ill families. It was felt that the almost inevitable frustration and discouragement of working with these families needed to be balanced by work with other families in which the likelihood of positive movement would be greater.

Thought was given to the type of agency or institution to which any future, similar program might be attached. Hospitals were thought to offer many advantages because patients turn there in times of crisis, and some families in the study showed indications of wanting to receive total services from this source. In view of the fact that most hospitals are not presently geared to offer outreaching services to families, it was suggested by the demonstration staff that mental health centers, welfare departments, child health clinics, and school services might be considered alternatives within which to locate such a program. Since many demonstration families seemed to require a social worker with authority, it was thought that a school department with a reaching-out type of service might be an effective locus. School departments would offer additional advantages in that children could be reached as early as kindergarten age and services could be offered in direct response to their needs. It was also thought that the community authority vested in a school representative would make it possible to focus on services to children without the necessity of having first to spend the time in meeting the mother's needs.

THE STUDY PEDIATRICIAN

The study pediatrician was a diplomate of the American Board of Pediatrics and, in addition, was a graduate of a school of public health. His previous experience covered work in hospitals, private practice, medical education, and public health.

Following the conclusion of his work with the Study he reported that it had provided an opportunity for the staff and himself to learn more about the health behavior of families with a multiplicity of problems. He felt, however, that the methods of health examination and evaluation employed in the Study were not transferable to a larger population. He noted that the cost in time and money was prohibitive and that the methods employed clearly could not be applied in a service program. He further suggested that screening examinations and evaluations of health needs for children, as pursued in the Study, would be of no value unless there were adequate follow-up and treatment resources available.

9

Implications of the Study

Since these studies have shown serious gaps in services for families with mentally ill parents, consideration should be given to ways whereby community services of health, education, and welfare might be strengthened to reduce unnecessary readmissions of parents to mental hospitals and emergency services, to help parents meet more adequately the needs of their children for child-care, and to assist the ill parent, expecially the mother, in efforts toward rehabilitation.

Needed Changes in Points of View

1) The first step toward improving services is to expand the point of view of those who are providing services as to what constitutes adequate or comprehensive care. In these studies the emphasis of most of the services was on the person as a mentally ill patient and least often on him as a parent of children. Often health and social services were unaware that the ill parent was concerned about the children and that this concern was aggravating the parent's illness. With a change in focus from one exclusively on the parent as a patient to a concern also for the parent as a member of a family and a caretaker, a clearer understanding of the total problems of the parent would result. Such an understanding would indicate those total problems in the patient's situation that are both contributing to his illness and affecting his family adversely. It would help to determine the best plan for the parent's care—whether to send him home from the emergency service if

he turned there for help or when to discharge him from the hospital and under what conditions. Thus, seeing the patient not only as a sick person but also as a spouse and parent within a family situation and living within a community would expand the knowledge of the parent as a patient and would give a clearer view of his total responsibilities and how they will affect and be affected by his illness. Without this point of view, services are likely to be limited and fractionated and followed by readmissions to mental hospitals.

2) Another point of view which bears examination is that the ill parent is the one who requires primary concern. The application of this point of view as shown in these studies resulted in the exposure of children to inadequate, even abusive care. This created problems for children, often serious in nature, as a result of which the services of other community agencies were required. This point of view also results in returning ill parents to their homes at serious costs to family members and to the very stability of the family itself rather than fully recognizing the hazards which are created in the family by the presence of the ill parent.

3) A current point of view of health and social agencies seems to be that the home is the best place for children regardless of the hazards involved. What separation of children from their homes and families really means to children and under what conditions needs to be scientifically examined and the limitations, both of care in the home and outside the home, carefully weighed. As demonstrated by these studies, supplementary care of children in order to protect them as well as to lessen the burdens on the ill mother has not generally been provided. Because of this emphasis on care of children by their mothers, more extended use of day care, whether in day care centers, day foster homes, or homes of relatives, friends, or neighbors, or foster care for the school week for preschool children, could relieve the pressures on the ill mother and the young children during the day when the older children are in school. This would make home care in their

own homes for the hours when they are there less traumatic both for the children and the ill parent. Controlled experiments should be instituted to test the values of such a system and to confirm or modify the present emphasis on care of children at home under almost all risks except in instances of legal neglect or abuse. Legislation should be expanded in order to protect children from the serious physical and psychological abuse resulting from a parent's mental illness.

4) The point of view is common which holds that no child should be placed away from home until all efforts have first been made to help the mother to become able to care for her children at home. In several families in these studies agencies had provided such help on a fractionated basis when crises occured, but the general welfare of some children, both physically and emotionally, was continuously inadequate. More effective services could be given to these families who are unable to provide a positive experience for children in their own homes by helping them to realize their limitations in providing a healthful enviornment for their children and supporting them in coming to the decision to have the children cared for elsewhere, either temporarily or permanently. A sharper analysis needs to be made earlier of the caretaking ability of parents. Such an analysis would permit a prognosis to be made as to the potential abilities of the parents to give adequate child-care. With such a careful evaluation, decisions could then justifiably be made about the kind of care children needed and steps could be taken with confidence to provide substitute care elsewhere when parents were considered to be unable to provide such themselves. At present, without this kind of study, parents unable to give adequate care to their children are pushed to try to do so, often making the situation worse for the children and the family. Some efforts in this direction were possible in the Study but only in cases of legal neglect or abuse. Others failed because of the points of view of most agencies that the child should stay in his own home, even with the problems therein, except for brief periods in acute situations. This point of view is being

tested elsewhere in a few studies. However, it merits further scientific investigation with controls in order to support or change the present emphases in most of our services which give little support to care away from home except in extreme cases of neglect.

5) The point of view that the mother's place is in the home rather than at work outside the home is being modified as the therapeutic value of work becomes clearer. In order, however, for the mother to work outside the home, she must have assistance in her usual home-care tasks. These studies showed that many mothers sought outside employment soon after they were discharged from the hospital, since they realized they were unable to cope with the situation at home and saw work as remedial. Thus the therapeutic use of outside employment for recuperating mentally ill mothers needs to be studied to determine the values, limitations, and the best timing for both mothers and children as well as thy supportive services needed in the home while the mother works. If points of view changed to be in favor of outside employment, home help services especially will need to be further developed to make such a plan possible and effective.

Day centers for mothers with built-in job training, medical and psychiatric services, and counseling would be very effective in helping some mothers to make the adjustment back into the community. Supportive services in the home would also be needed to make such a plan feasible.

6) The point of view, also still held by most health and social agencies, that the services are better utilized if the individual is motivated to seek them out and actually applies for help was not validated in this Study. Families of hospitalized parents graciously welcomed the offer of services when the agency's representative went to their homes to express interest in helping them with plans for the care of their children and in the problems in the family caused by the parent's illness. Families verbally expressed appreciation for what they recognized as an unusual method of offering help. They were even more

motivated to make use of the services and noticeably followed through in many instances. Thus a change in the point of view that the individual must, on his own volition, be motivated to apply for agency services, either for health or social needs, was not supported in these studies. This suggests with mentally ill parents, especially since their illness naturally prevents many of them from seeking help, that services are needed which will reach out to them and lessen their embarrassment in volunteering that they have a mentally ill member in the family. Reaching out to offer services has applicability to health as well as social services and could result in providing more mental health care in the patient's own home or at least in neighborhood centers. Availability of psychiatric and social services in the home in an emergency might result in finding families with mental illness before the illness reaches the acute stage. Such a home service for acute episodes of mental illness has been found very effective in Amsterdam. It could eventually be a part of a proposed plan for neighborhood health and welfare centers.

7) Similarly the point of view about priorities in providing services may need to be further considered. Many agencies consider their first priority must be to give care to the sick who recognize that they are sick or to those families that seek help. When the sick are cared for, as a second priority, agencies could consider providing care to those not so acutely in need. At present agencies usually have no time, staff, or funds left to provide services to those less acutely in need. Emphasis on preventive measures would result in giving services to the less acutely ill also as well as to the needs of others in the family. Thus, a change in point of view which emphasizes the importance of preventive measures as well as curative services would change both the focus and extent of our health and welfare services. To treat one member of the family while the spouse and children continue to be seriously affected by the sick member does little to decrease the incidence of health and social problems. It adds to the increasing number of individuals and families who need treatment to the point that the capacities of the agencies are

inadequate to provide the needed care. With conviction about the need to reduce the incidence and with clarification of the ways to do so, the incidence could probably be lessened.

8) The point of view that only services which are aimed at treating the basic psychological problems in a family are of any real or lasting consequence is slowly changing in the direction of placing value on external supports. However, in these studies there was little evidence that external props had been used to any degree. The limited use of such supplementary services as home-helps, day-care services, summer camps, after-school programs for children, vacation for parents, time away from home for the ill parent to work or play, guidance in homemaking, strengthened church ties, and others were very infrequently used and then not usually in any imaginative way. More emphasis placed on those opportunities which will provide the ill parent with some of the positive experiences in life rather than burdening him with overpowering parental responsibilities while still sick would prove beneficial both to the ill parent and the family, especially the children.

This point of view that only treatment of the basic psychological problem is effective was apparent when ill mothers refused psychiatric services or were unable to discuss their emotional problems with the social workers. Then there was a tendency on the part of psychiatrists and social workers to believe that the patient was "inaccessible to treatment." Perhaps one way of helping a mother to be more "accessible" would be to free her from some of the realistic burdens and strains that were so prevalent in these families. To do this effectively will require a change in point of view which emphasizes the therapeutic value of these supports and which provides for their use through expanded resources. However, more use could be made of normal resources, such as relatives, friends, libraries, schools, and churches, already available to families. Perhaps too often the tendency is to turn for help to organized sources that are already overburdened and cannot provide the same kind of natural, informal props as the normal resources can provide nor for as continuous a period of time.

9) Agencies need to change their point of view in regard to what can be expected of mentally ill parents, especially mothers, in a relatively short time. In this study, psychiatric and social agencies tended to be discouraged because progress toward resolution of problems was slow and many times work with the families was terminated too early. The efforts of the demonstration workers have shown that these families were not able to change in a limited time because they had basic difficulties in facing their own needs and those within their families and in accepting the fact that something needed to be done. Parents vascillated in their readiness to move ahead and time was needed to help them before they were ready to take the necessary steps for themselves or their children. If progress is to be made with these families with severe deficits in family functioning, psychiatric and social agencies will need to accept the fact that long-time, continuous support and guidance of a fairly direct nature is needed. Students preparing to work with such families, either in the health or social agencies, will need to be taught the different techniques required for this kind of service and to develop skills in the use of external supports which may require further development to meet the needs. Imaginative utilization of existing services and skill in improvising a needed program to help families improve their abilities to function adequately are essential in these families already overcome by the multiplicity of the problems in which they are entrenched.

10) Another point of view that limits the effectiveness of our present services is the belief that agencies belong primarily to the client and therefore they are responsible to the client to provide what he wants and what the agency believes he needs. This responsibility to the client is considered to supersede the agency's responsibility to other agencies and through them to the community. The point of view is still unusual that organized services are provided for families in the community as a network of services, each with its special function. An agency is

dependent on other agencies to contribute to the total needs in families with many problems. Without such interagency relationships, a fractionated program results. Some agencies often refuse to share their knowledge of the family situation with other services for the purpose of working together toward better care for the individual or family. The extreme application of the principle of confidentiality, which permits little if any real sharing with other agencies, contributes to this lack of coordination and joint planning, and sometimes results in conflicting advice that causes serious confusion for the family. Clearer thinking needs to be done in regard to the individual's or family's expectations of what is involved in agency services in order to evaluate this point of view. Certainly most families expect the health and social agencies to make the best use of other resources for their welfare and trust the agencies to work together in the best interests of the family. This point of view is perhaps more crucial in relation to the individual who is mentally ill than in relation to other persons since the mentally ill person is often less able to make such a judgment and may also be more defensive about discussing his mental illness with non-psychiatric agencies.

Expansion or Reorganization of Services

The points of view previously discussed serve as some of the foundations on which programs and policies are developed within our community services. They are, therefore, basic to any consideration of expansion or reorganization of services.

Immediate Steps

Some essential steps that must be taken immediately to alleviate the serious impact of mental illness on children are as follows:

1) Health and social agencies should require their staffs, who are working with individuals or families, to broaden their study of the family situation to determine what individuals in the family seem to be presenting symptoms of mental illness and the number and age of any children in the family. After identification of the ill person and the children, the staff member could then be required to see that the ill person and the children received the help they needed by providing services directly through his own agency or by referral to appropriate resources. To leave these needs unattended should be against the policies of all agencies.

2) Mental hospitals could readily identify parents who have children at home by adding these items to the admitting face sheets. Inquiry could then be made by the hospital social workers regarding the family's need for help in planning for the care of children during the parent's hospitalization and in working with the other parent or relatives in relation to problems within the family. If social work service were focused at the point of admission and services provided during the patient's hospitalization, families would be more likely to be ready for the patient's return. Also, better planning would result and the ill parent would be relieved by knowing about the plan for the care of the children during his hospitalization. The social worker at admission, if time permitted, could then help families with child-care problems or could refer the family to the appropriate agency in the community, probably either a mental health center or a family agency. The agency, by agreement with the hospital, could immediately offer services to these families to assist them in making arrangements for adequate child-care which would continue as long as necessary. This agency would then work closely with the social worker in the hospital so that planning for the patient and the family could be integrated.

3) In order to provide the necessary supplementary services for children in their own homes, most communities need an expansion of day-care services which will provide care for full days or parts of a day

and sometimes to care for school children before and after school hours and at lunch time. This care could then be fitted into the parent's hours of employment. For children of hospitalized mothers who need care when the fathers' work hours are different from the hours of the day-care center, day foster-home care for them and for infants needs to be developed either to be used on a daily basis or for 24 hour care during the period of the fathers' employment or for longer periods of time. These services could be used effectively also for children of mentally ill mothers who are at home.

4) Day centers for parents recuperating from an acute mental illness or as a preventative to a mental crisis need to be available as a means of helping the parent to separate from the hospital, to fit into a group in the community, and to provide continuity in the medical and psychiatric care of the parent. Job training and preparation for returning to work, whether at home or in the community, should be an important part of the program. Services of the various professions would be required since the emphasis is on rehabilitation in all aspects of functioning.

5) Home-help and homemaker services need to be expanded. When available, they could be used to keep a family intact while the ill mother is hospitalized or to assist the ill mother on a full- or part-time basis when she is at home. Flexibility in hours so as to fit into the family's needs are essential as well as continuity of services for as long as needed.

6) Extension of psychiatric services into the homes of many of these families would have provided continuity in psychiatric care and would have given the psychiatrist a clearer picture of the ill parent's home situation. The psychiatrist would then be more able to participate realistically in planning with the community agencies for the needs of the family. Psychiatric services available for home care would also be more effective in mental crises since planning for care could be done in relation to the family's situation and with greater knowledge of the needs of members of the family.

7) If emergency psychiatric care is to continue to be given through emergency services of general hospitals, the pattern used in one general hospital in the Study seemed to have good potentials for providing care. The staff consisted of the usual psychiatric team. The emergency service was staffed throughout the 24 hours. The major limitations seemed to be in the imcomplete understanding of the home situation, and the decision to return the parent immediately to the home without direct knowledge of what this could mean to the patient or the family, especially the children. Also, the lack of any real follow-up program, other than to advise the patient to return, usually resulted in interrupted service. Furthermore, few parents were referred to community agencies to provide help with problems or needs in the family even though the emergency service did not assume responsibility for providing such service itself. If the hospital does not provide the social work services needed, it would be well, in order to assess the family situation and the problems of the ill parent and family members, to refer the family to a community agency, such as a mental health center, for evaluation of the family situation, follow-up of the patient and assistance with the problems of child-care. If there is no mental health center, agreements might be drawn up between the hospital and a community agency, such as a family service or public health nursing agency, to locate families and to refer them to appropriate agencies for service.

8) There was lack of coordination between the schools and the health and social agencies even when the schools recognized that problems existed in the homes of many children which affected the children's school program. This suggests again that some plan of collaboration between the schools and the health and social agencies working with the families is necessary in order that health and social agencies may be more aware of the impact of the parent's mental illness on the child as shown through the child's school experiences and in order to plan with the school so that the school can help in lessening the impact of the

parent's illness on the child. More adequate school social work services, closely related to the health services of the school and working with health and social agencies in the community, would make this possible.

Reorganization of Services

The main emphasis in the previous discussion was on the inseparability of the mentally ill parent and his social situation. This implies that the patient cannot be treated in a vacuum, whether the vacuum is the emergency service or the mental hospital, for the patient brings with him not only his life's experiences in the past, but also his present situation which involves his spouse, his children, his family as a unit, his relatives and friends, his job, and other ties and responsibilities. Whatever services attempt to help him to be effective must not only consider these identifications, but must also involve them, either directly or through the patient or his representative, in a plan for the patient's future. These studies have shown that there was not such comprehensive consideration and planning in the services and that, as a result, patients received too little psychiatric and social services for too short a time and on too individualized a basis. Also, the studies showed that other community services working with the patient, even at the same time, were in no way related to each other in their efforts. Therefore, some plan which is consistent, allows for coordination, and which provides ongoing services on the part of one or more agencies is essential for adequate care to families with mental illness.

Ideally gaps and duplications in services could be avoided if one agency assumed an ongoing relationship with the patient and provided the coordination of services when other agencies were also involved with the family. In these studies it was found that, in general, except in the demonstration cases, no agencies assumed such a coordinating role. Without it there were gaps and inconsistencies in services and duplications in treatment efforts, resulting in confusion for the family.

In the demonstration in Study II a community coordinating committee of representatives of health, education, and the social services was formed which served as a committee responsible to reach out to provide services to all families with a parent hospitalized in a mental hospital. The committee, therefore, took on a community responsibility to see that services were given immediately and for as long a period as was needed. This plan worked well; its limitations were primarily due to the pressures of other responsibilities which limited the extent and duration of the services. However, the plan merits application. There could be in each area a coordinating committee of representatives of health, education, and the social services, which would be responsible for planning the coordination of those community services that agreed to coordinate their efforts with other agencies in an attempt to provide a program of comprehensive and continuous care and supervision to these families. The pattern of continuous supervision and follow-up has been well established in health planning for crippled children and for families with tuberculosis. Such a pattern might well be utilized for families with mentally ill parents. It would mean that clinical services, social agencies, and the schools concerned with the children's progress would follow through to provide services whenever needed for the care of the patient or problems within the family and to meet the needs of children.

An ideal organizational plan to meet these problems would be as follows. In the further development of community centers all health and social services, both public and voluntary, might be included to form a unified center, not just a group of coordinated agencies. The center would be responsible to the community to help families with whatever problems they knew about or which were identified by others, such as the schools, churches, private physicians, and employers. Families would perceive these centers as established in their community for them and they would participate in decisions regarding policies and programs. They would thus come to have confidence and trust in the center and would be expected to turn more readily to the staff for advice. Neighbors, friends, and relatives would know the center and would readily share with the center the knowledge of problems of families in the community which they felt needed help. Through those staff members of the center who frequently visited families for other purposes, such as physicians, public health nurses, social workers, especially from welfare programs, and sanitarians, any situation in which a problem of mental illness was suspected would be discussed with the mental health division and the appropriate steps determined according to the severity of the problem. Persons would be referred when necessary to hospitals through the staffs of these centers. There would be one family record to which each staff member working with the family would contribute. Thus, fractionization by individual, illness, age, location, or type of service would be avoided. Through planning conferences within the staff, an assessment of the problems within the family would be made as well as decisions as to what staff members could assume the responsibility for providing the services. One staff member would be assigned as the coordinator of the services for a given family in order to assure that the needed services were provided in an integrated manner. He would be responsible for calling subsequent conferences for planning purposes when necessary. If more than one service were needed, the coordinator would clarify with the family the roles of each and their purposes. Thus, a unified approach would be made to the solution of the family's problems, avoiding gaps and duplications in services. When certain staff members completed their work, the rest of the staff involved would know this because this would be a joint decision. In these studies an agency often assumed that another agency was still working with the family—even though the other agency had closed its case some time before, leaving a gap in the continuity of care. It would be hoped that there would be general oversight by the coordinator through visits to the home after the specialized services had been completed until the family seemed to be able to manage on its own with a fair degree of success. Planned follow-up with the family would be essential in order to identify new or recurrent problems in their incipiency.

This Study indicates that only some kind of continuous and integrated program of service focused on the whole family and its problems can meet the varied and multiple needs in most families with mentally ill parents.

Whatever the organizational pattern, consideration should be given to the problems of the patient in his family; to the needs of the family members—especially the children—affected by the patient's illness; to ways of providing consistant and continuous care; and to the need for coordination of all community services working with the family. The extensiveness and severity of problems existing in families when there is a parent with mental illness requires broad and cooperative community planning of health, education, and welfare without which many children will be unprotected and little progress made in the rehabilitation of mentally ill parents. Without such an approach to the numerous and varied problems often present in families with mental illness, there will be little reduction in the incidence of such problems which seriously affect the community, the family, and each individual child.

In most cases communtiy agencies of health, education, and welfare had failed for the most part over the years to provide the services required to help these families to function responsibly or to provide the kind of care children needed for their healthy development. As a result many children were exposed to hazards in their environment, resulting in emotional or social distrubances which will inevitably require help from health and social services in the future at an inestimable cost to the community and at a great sacrifice of potential strengths to the children themselves. The problem is clear; its solution requires immediate, united planning by health, education, and social services.

10

Summary

The extent and severity of risk created for children when one of their parents is mentally ill have received little attention in the past. A few studies have presented some aspects of the impact of parental mental illness on children. The three studies reported in this volume have described the impact on 652 children whose mentally ill parents were hospitalized in a state mental hospital or were seen in an emergency psychiatric service of one of two general hospitals. A small number of parents hospitalized in two public sanatoria were included in the pilot study in order to determine if there were any major differences in the child-caretaking plans when a patient's hospitalization was for a physical rather than a mental illness. Although the proportions of families with children separated from their own homes were similar in both the physically and mentally hospitalized parents, there were other factors that increased the disruption and distress of children of mentally ill parents. The later studies, therefore, concerned only mentally ill parents and their children. Fathers who were patients were included in the first two studies but not in the third because the mental illness of mothers was found to have more impact on children and the problems of child-care.

No black families were included in the first two studies since there were none who met the two criteria definitions of age and children living in the home. This reflected the smaller proportion of black families living in small towns and suburban areas than in urban areas. In Study III, in an urban area, about a fourth of the mothers were black.

The first two studies included families of a parent hospitalized who lived in the small towns or suburban areas served by the cooperating hospitals while the third study drew its families from a large urban area with several areas of marked socioeconomic deprevation.

The Study Design

The pilot study (Study I) showed that, in general, families did not receive help from the hospital in planning for the care of their children when a parent was hospitalized and did not generally turn to community agencies for such assistance on their own volition. The following two studies, therefore, were planned as demonstration studies in which services were built into the study design. In the second study families living in two small cities became the demonstration families while families in thirteen towns served by the hospital were the control families. In the demonstration cities, community agencies, which were often used to help in planning for families and children, were organized, with the help of the study staff, into Community Committees to which families were referred by the Study's case finder located in the mental hospital. Immediately after referral the family was then assigned, by the coordinator of the community committee, to one of the agencies for study and assistance with the understanding that each agency would reach out to offer services to the family and would keep in close touch with the families during the study year in order to assess the number and severity of problems and to help with any existing difficulties. The control families in the small towns received no assistance instigated by the Study staff but used only those resources that they sought on their own volition.

Because the demonstration workers in Study II did not, in most instances, maintain regular and consistent relationships with the study families during all of the study year, due in part to pressures of their regular responsibilities to other families in the community, demonstration workers were added in Study III as a part of the Study staff in order to ensure that they would be free to provide continuous and preventive services needed throughout the study year.

Research interviewers in all three studies used a semistructured schedule in their home interviews with parents, relatives, or other caretakers. In the first two studies, since the ill parent was hospitalized, the interviews were usually with other caretakers than the ill parent, while in the third study, in which most of the ill mothers were at home following their visits to emergency psychiatric services, the interviews were with the ill mother. Two research interviews were completed within a 6-month period in the first study while three interviews over the period of 1 year were carried out in the other two studies. The data from these interviews, the reports of the demonstration workers, school reports, reports of community agencies which had known the families during the study year, and reports from health agencies served as the basis for the findings reported in this volume. In addition, in the third study, the reports of two examinations of children and the recommendations of the pediatrician, a member of the Study staff, provided more uniform, consistent, and comprehensive data on the children's physical and emotional status.

The three studies in sequence were completed between 1959 and 1967. The total number of families with ill parents were 253 with 652 children.

THE ILL PARENTS

Of the 253 ill parents, 225 were mentally ill and 28 were parents with tuberculosis; 199 were mothers and 54 were fathers. Of the 199 mothers, 74 (32%) were one-parent families. The urban study (Study III) had the highest proportion (46%) of mothers of one-parent families.

The presenting problems of the mentally ill parents were categorized into (1) presenting problems related to children, and (2) presenting problems related to the emotional or psychiatric symptoms of the ill parent. Problems of parents related to children included abuse, neglect and fear of harming children, worry about children, parent-child conflicts, difficulties in coping with the care of children, and difficulties related to unwanted pregnancies or births. Problems in these areas were reported by 42% of the mentally ill mothers and 12% of the mentally ill fathers.

Presenting problems related to the parents' emotional or psychiatric symptoms were identified among 76% of the mentally ill mothers and 60% of the mentally ill fathers. These symptoms included delusional or hallucinatory symptoms, suicidal attempts, gestures or impulses, and other affective or somatic complaints. Thus the majority of ill parents reported problems of this nature; the distress and disruption which these problems caused for children were vividly described in the research interviews and the records of the demonstration workers. These symptoms, furthermore, were often of long duration: the proportion of patients with symtoms lasting 6 months or more ranged from 23.5% to as high as 44.5%, indicating that these problems were not acute.

Of the mentally ill parents hospitalized in Studies I and II over half had had prior admissions to a mental hospital while around a quarter of the parents seen in the emergency psychiatric services in Study III had had prior care in a mental hospital. The proportion of mothers in one-parent families who had had previous care in a mental hospital was greater in Study I than for ill parents in two-parent families. However, this was reversed in the other two studies.

As might be expected, the ill parents hospitalized in Studies I and II had a higher proportion with psychotic diagnosed illness while the ill mothers seen in the emergency psychiatric services had a higher proportion with psychoneurotic conditions. Even during the study year, 25% of ill parents had been readmitted to the hospital, thus creating another upsetting experience for children.

THE FAMILIES

The families in the three studies were described by selected demographic characteristics. The ill fathers were generally older than the ill mothers; the mothers in one-parent families were younger than mothers in two-parent families; and mothers in Study III, the urban study, were younger than those in the other two studies. Mothers hospitalized for tuberculosis in Study I were younger than the mentally ill mothers. The control mothers in Study III were somewhat older than demonstration mothers.

The proportion of one-parent families in the studies was considerably greater than the proportion of one-parent families in the Boston Metropolitan Area. Mothers of one-parent families in Study III, especially black mothers, had been separated from their husbands for a longer period of time than in the other studies. When the parents had been separated for less than a month, the crises associated with separation were frequently followed by the parents' hospitalization.

The religious affiliation of the white families was predominantly Catholic in all of these studies and the proportion of Catholic families exceeded that of the Boston Metropolitan Area. The black families in Study III, however, were more frequently Protestant. There were few Jewish families or families of other religions.

The educational attainment of the ill mothers was lower than that of the Boston Metropolitan Area in Studies I and III. Black mothers had the lowest educational attainment.

One-parent families had lower incomes than two-parent families. This was also true of urban families as contrasted with the families in small towns and suburban areas. Also black families in Study III had smaller incomes than white families.

The modal occupation of the fathers, both ill and well, was that of operative or laborer. The husbands of ill mothers in the urban study were more frequently unemployed and had held their jobs for shorter periods of time than those in the other studies. Black fathers had held their jobs for shorter periods of time than white fathers; they had the highest proportion of unemployment and the lowest proportion of regular employment during the study year.

One-parent families had moved more frequently than two-parent families and black families more than whites. Also one-parent families owned their own homes less frequently than two-parent families and were particularly vulnerable to the loss of their home following the parent's hospitalization. In the urban study, especially in one-parent families, housing conditions were characterized by overcrowding, poor housekeeping, slum conditions, multiple family homes, and housing projects.

Ill fathers differed from husbands of ill mothers in that they received less imcome, held their jobs for shorter periods, were more frequently unemployed, and were more often dependent on the income from the mother's employment. Their families were more mobile, owned their own homes less frequently, and were more frequently receiving public assistance.

Mothers in Study III had had more pregnancies than mothers in the other studies: black mothers had the highest mean number of pregnancies. Fetal death rates were higher for two-parent families, but not for one-parent families in Study III than in the other studies and were highest of all among the black two-parent families in Study III. Among families with ill mothers, the mean number of study children per family was greater in Study III than in the other studies. The two-parent families in all three studies and the one-parent families in

Study III had as many as four children more often than did the population of the Boston Metropolitan Area.

The largest number of children under 18 years of age not living at home was in Study III. Most of these children were in two-parent families. The largest proportion of them were placed in foster homes under supervision of the public child welfare agency, while the next largest group lived with relatives.

THE CHILDREN

In families with mentally ill parents the children were variously involved in the emotional disturbances and the distressing and upsetting experiences that occurred in the home. Some children were intimately and seriously involved in the bizarre symptoms of their parents while others seemed unaware of the illness. The data reporting the experiences of the children were obtained in the research interviews with the fathers of caretakers in the first two studies and with the ill mothers at home in the third study. When the fathers were hospitalized the mothers reported about the children. Therefore there were some differences in the responses and some negative experiences were withheld in an effort by the respondent to minimize or deny the extent of the mental illness. In Study III the mentally ill mothers at home were not questioned about the impact on children of their own mental illness for they were either too emotionally unstable to be able to give dependable answers or were threatened by such questions, fearing their children would be taken away.

The children were classified into two groups: (1) those who were upset by the illness, or (2) those children who were neglected or abused. It was interesting that among the control families with a turberculous parent in Study I only a few mothers reported their children were upset because of their illness and hospitalization while the families of ill fathers reported that no child was upset because of the illness. Also in none of the families with a tuberculous parent was there any report of neglect or abuse of children. The time factor before the tuberculous parent was admitted to the sanatorium allowed the parents to plan for substitute child-care and to give the children explanations of the illness and need for hospitalization.

A higher proportion of children of mentally ill parents were involved in the parents' symptomatology then in the case of tuberculous parents. Also there were more reports of neglect and abuse of children of mentally ill parents. These reports were greater in the urban study than in the two previous studies in small towns and suburban areas. Parents of some children reported that the children cried more than usual and seemed sad. Others were upset at the violent and uncontrollable behavior of the sick parent; some mothers expected their children to care for them; and other children mimicked or assumed symptoms of the ill parent. Some children were abused by their mothers; others bitten, beaten, or threatened with knives. Almost half of the families in Studies II and III reported mistreatment of children. Other children were frightened by the parents' behavior or suicidal attempts. Some children begged that the ill parent be hospitalized and others showed relief when the ill parent was out of the home.

Involvement of the children in the symptoms of the ill parent was reported in over half of the families in all three studies, ranging from 55 to 80% of the families. Almost half of the families with mentally ill fathers also reported involvement of the children in the parental illness. The involvement of the children in the symptoms of the parents' illness ranged from relatively minor, upsetting incidents to grave traumatic experiences of serious impact when the children showed confusion, bewilderment, fright, sadness, or experienced unprovoked beatings or outright abuse resulting in physical injuries. Even in families which reported "no involvement" of the children in the illness of the parent, there were indications that these reports were not correct. The reports of no involvement were usually in relation to children under 6 years.

The difficulties of children as reported in the research interviews were separated into behavioral difficulties and neurotic traits. Over half of the children were reported to have none of these types. The proportion of children with these difficulties was higher in families with mentally ill parents than in families with tuberculous parents. The behavioral difficulties ranged from ones of a minor or transient nature to those of serious proportions. They included management problems, temper tantrums, excessive shyness, or delinquent acts. The highest proportion of children with neurotic difficulties were reported to be "nervous." Other neurotic traits included nail-biting, enuresis, eating or sleeping difficulties, headaches, and fears. Somewhat more children were reported to have neurotic traits than behavioral difficulties. The children of mentally ill fathers had the highest proportion of reported neurotic traits.

School

Over two-thirds of the children in the study with school reports were at the usual grade for their age; 17% were below grade and 15% were above grade average. Slightly over one-quarter of the children had repeated school grades. Of children who had repeated grades a slightly higher proportion were in families with mentally ill parents than in families with tuberculous parents. Also there was a higher proportion among children of two-parent families than one-parent families. More black children in Study III had repeated grades than white children.

Children in one-parent families seemed to have a better academic record than children in two-parent families. They had a higher proportion of children above grade and at grade level and a lower proportion below grade. These differences may be due in part to the problems in the homes of two-parent families in which severe marital discord was reported in almost half. In Study III these differences between children of one- and two-parent families were even clearer: the average age of the children was the same yet the children of one-parent families were a grade higher in school than the children of two-parent families. Children of one-parent families also had fewer repeated grades and fewer of them were reported by their teachers to be not well adjusted. Also teachers reported fewer to have difficulties in their home conditions including problems of child-care.

Three-fifths of the children with above average academic standing, although doing well in their grades, were reported by the schools to have behavioral difficulties or problems of absence. The problems within the family situation were often coexistent with difficulties in the child's behavior at school, showing the relation of the home situation to the child's school behavior. The most common behavioral difficulty reported by the teachers of these children with above average academic standing was that the child was withdrawn; a few were aggressive or disruptive in the classroom.

The behavioral difficulties reported most frequently by the teachers were neurotic tendencies. This group included the larger number of children and the larger number of problems per child. These may have been more frequent because of the relatively over-all young average age of the children, 8 years. There were few high school children in the study; a few who had dropped out of school at 16 years had shown serious aggressive, delinquent-type behavior.

Over a quarter of the children were reported by the schools to have limitations in sight, hearing, speech, or motor activity which interfered with their expected academic achievement. In addition, teachers expressed concern with over half of the children because of frequent absences, poor motivation, personality and behavioral difficulties, or home and health problems. The teachers considered nearly two-thirds of the children able to do better academic work. In only a quarter of the children had the school had contact with the parents about any problem.

Efforts of the demonstration workers in Study III were primarily focused on problems in the home situations and the care of children rather than on the children's school cifficulites. They pointed out, however, that the schools had an unusual opportunity to identify problems of children and together with other community agencies to work toward the alleviation and prevention of problems of children of mentally ill parents. The incidence and severity of problems of children require concerted and collaborative effort on the part of community health, education and welfare programs.

The Health of Children

Information about the health problems and the medical resources used was secured from the families in Studies I and II. In Study III the data was obtained from the two examinations made early in the study year and at the end of the year by the pediatrician on the study staff.

In Studies I and II the most frequent health resource used by families was the services of private physicians. For the children of tuberculous parents, local health deparement clinics for contact examinations and hospital outpatient departments were used more frequently than in the demonstration families with mentally ill parents.

In Study I no health problems were reported by the caretakers for 64% of the children and in Study II for 74% of the children. In Study III the health history taken by the pediatrician showed nearly half of the 177 children had a history of at least one accident and one admission to a hospital. 28% had frequent illnesses and 16% were reported by the pediatrician to have retarded development or learning. The most common health problems in all three studies had been difficulties with vision. Frequent colds and speech problems in Study II, allergies in Studies I and II, and difficulties with urinary conditions or genitalia in Study III were the health problems second highest in number. Allergies, and visual difficulties were reported most among children 6 years and over and frequent colds in children under 6, especially those under three. During the study year, respiratory infections and accidents were the most common health problems reported. There was a high rate of hospitalization of children during the study year. In Study I this reflected the susceptibility to tuberculosis of children in the control group. Other hospitalizations were mostly for accidents or acute medical or surgical problems. Where hospital rates were especially high among children under 6 years of age in Study III, a quarter of the children under 6 had no health supervision while a fifth over 6 had none. The most frequent sources of health supervision in Study III were the child health clinics of the city sometimes combined with the school health services. Inadequate health supervision was more frequently reported for children from one-parent and black families. Black one-parent children had the least health supervision. A somewhat higher proportion of children at the end of the study year had had health supervision as a result of the recommendations of the Study pediatrician.

Most of the children in this urban study, as would be expected, received their medical care from the city hospital clinics sometimes supplemented by other resources. Few children of one-parent families and only one black child had private physicians.

In Study III over a fifth of the 177 children, including 68% of those under 3 years of age, had not completed their basic immunizations at the time of the first examination by the Study's pediatrician. Children of one-parent and black families were again less well protected. By the time of the second examination there was an improvement in immunization status for both demonstration and control families which was ascribed to the initial pediatric recommendations for both groups.

The most frequent health need found by the pediatrician was for dental care; in approximately half of the children 3 years or over dental care was needed soon or urgently. There was no over-all marked improvement in dental need at the time of the second examination.

Nearly half of the children had a history of one accident or one hospitalization. Frequent illnesses and accidents were reported more often for children under 6 years, especially black children, than for children over 6 years. Also black children in the older age group had had at least one accident more frequently than white children. Hospitalization was reported to be more frequent among school-aged children than preschool children. The rate of hospitalization of children during the study year was higher than the rate in recent national health surveys.

Health problems for which medical treatment had not been obtained prior to the pediatric examination were those of vision; bones, joints, or muscles; ear, nose, and throat; heart; kindey, bladder, or genitalia; hernia; and nutrition. In most instances the families had known about the conditions but had secured no medical care for them. Conditions more frequently unknown to the family included heart conditions and those related to the lungs, blood conditions, and hernias.

A larger proportion of black than white children were given an over-all health rating of *good* at the time of the first pediatric examination. By the second examination the proportion who showed improvement in their health rating was somewhat larger than the proportion whose rating was poorer. These ratings were similar for both demonstration and control families.

By the time of the second examination families had failed to take action on the pediatric recommendations in the cases of only 15% of the children (26 of 177 children). This failure occurred significantly more frequently in black two-parent families than in white two-parent families, but black one-parent families had a significantly larger proportion who followed through on the pediatric recommendations that white one-parent families. Families with less than four children followed the recommendation more frequently than families with four or more children. Also children under 6 received more attention than older children.

The response to the recommendations of the pediatrician was

widespread in the study families. The most frequent reason given by the families for not following through on the recommendations was that they did not consider the recommendations important; less frequently they complained of the cost of care or that the parent was too busy.

PROVISIONS FOR CARE

When a parent showed symptoms of mental illness for a shorter or longer period of time there were often many distressful and disruptive effects on children. In some cases the ill parents had shown disturbed behavior for some time but the need for treatment had been unrecognized, delayed, or denied by them and their families. In these families it was often a relief for the other parent and the children when the ill parent was hospitalized. Thus for some time children had usually been exposed to these disruptive episodes in their homes which in many cases were only brought to light at the time of hospitalization when substitute care for children was needed. Thus some method of helping these families before the parent becomes so ill that hospitalization is required is essential if children are to be protected from the risks resulting from their exposure to the mental illness of a parent in the home. Even identification of these children at the point when the parent, in an acute episode, seeks care in an emergency service is too late to lessen the impact on children of the experiences with a mentally ill parent which have been building up for months, sometimes years.

When the parent was hospitalized there were usually problems of obtaining the care for the children. This was especially so when the mother was the parent hospitalized for the children were frequently separated from their own homes. This was true of the children with mothers in hospitals for either mental illness or tuberculosis. In contrast, when the fathers were hospitalized there was relatively little disruption in the living arrangements or care of children who usually remained in their own homes with their mothers. In a very few families the fathers had already been separated from the family before admission; these separations were usually due to marital difficulties involved in the father's mental illness. In almost half of these families with ill fathers the mothers had worked outside their homes prior to the fathers' hospitalization and continued to do so after the fathers' admissions. For the children in these families, therefore, no additional or different child-care problems arose.

When parents were hospitalized the children had the same types of risks as other children whose fathers or mothers were absent from the home because of separation, divorce, death, or other reasons. In addition they also had the risk of having a parent who was ill for a shorter or longer period of time and was hospitalized. Because of the uncertainties about the duration of hospital stay, planning for substitute care of these children was made more difficult for the family.

Separations from their own homes often resulted also in separations from the other parent, siblings, peers, their regular school, or the familiarity of their own neighborhood and community. Thus often through separation the child was away from all that was familiar to him and for an uncertain period of time. Three factors consistently determined the extent of the disruptions: (1) the hospitalization of the mother caused considerably more disruption in the living arrangements and care of the children that the hospitalization of the father; (2) the children of one-parent families with ill mothers experienced the greatest disruption since children were then left without a parent; and (3) families varied from those with adequate resources to care for children to those with few or no resources to care for children. In these studies, when mothers were hospitalized, separation of children from their own homes occurred in just under one-third of the two-parent families but in about two-thirds of the one-parent families. This was true both in the families with mentally ill parents and in those with tuberculous parents. However, there were interesting differences between these two groups due to several advantages that the families of tuberculous parents had which were not true of the families with mentally ill parents such as: (1) a period of time to prepare for hospitalization; (2) an anticipated, approximate length of hospitalization; (3) a longer period of hospitalization but few readmissions; and (4) a greater acceptance by the family and the patients of the need for hospitalization, as contrasted with strong resistance to hospitalization by the mentally ill parent and often of his family.

The resources within the family largely determined whether children were separated from their homes. Resources frequently used were: (1) a relative living in the home or available to come to the home; (2) older children in the family who cared for themselves and sometimes assumed major or total care of the younger children; (3) friends, neighbors, or baby sitters; and (4) paid help or homemaker services. Without these resources children were usually separated from home. They were most often sent to homes of relatives but a few had foster-home or institutional placements. The demonstration workers influenced the plan for child-care in a few families either by providing homemaker services so that children could stay at home or by arranging care away from home in some families when the home situation for some time had been injurious to children.

When mothers were readmitted to the hospital, as happened in almost one-fourth of the mentally ill mothers during the study year, it was often more difficult and complicated to make plans for children because relatives frequently were unwilling to take the children again. Relatives tended to return the children to their homes as soon as the mothers arrived home from the hospital. It is probable that the assumption of full responsibilities by the mother so soon after hospitalization contributed to the need for subsequent hospital care.

Separations of children also occurred in a fifth of the families for reasons other than the hospitalization of the mother. These separations were largely the result of the ill mother's inability to cope with the care of the children when she was at home. In some families the mother-child relationships and the distress associated with the mother's mental illness were so disturbing that the child was seriously exposed to the emotional or physical strains involved. Young children up to 2 years of age were the ones placed most often. The preschool children were the ones most difficult for relatives to care for indefinitely. Shifting about of the children among the relatives occured frequently. The number of shifts varied from one shift to as many as seven in the study year. This meant that siblings were often separated.

Older children sometimes separated themselves from the family because of the difficulties under which they had been living in the home with the ill parent. Some went to live permanently with relatives or friends while others moved away or entered into early and uncertain marriages.

Children in one-parent families with an ill mother had the highest frequency of separation and this was true whether the mothers were hospitalized or ill at home. Among one-parent families with ill mothers, this ranged from a half to over four-fifths of the children. In contrast in two-parent families only a third of the children experienced separation, and these were mostly the younger children. The most vulnerable groups of children from the point of view of separation were those under 2 years of age and the preschool group in one-parent families with mothers ill or hospitalized.

Similarly the younger children presented the greatest child-care problems even in their own homes for they required continuous care and supervision whereas the older children were in school a large part of the time. The care provided to children in their own homes was not always desirable or harmonious. This was often the case when the ill mother was in the home but also true of some substitute caretakers. Sometimes the older children were responsible for the care of the smaller ones or rather hit-or-miss arrangements were made for part-time child-care. This was more true of two-parent families in which the father took over the child-care when he returned from work.

The variety, extent, and complications involved in the arrangements for substitute care of children ranged from relatively simple, easily made, and sympathetically arranged plans to highly complicated, inadequate, fragmented, or multiple care plans.

Employment of mothers also added another problem in child-care. Over a third of the mothers were employed sometime during the study year. The proportion was higher for one-parent than for two-parent families and considerably higher when the fathers were ill. In over half of these families the children were under school age and were cared for by relatives, neighbors, or older children, or in two-parent families fathers carried this role for the time the mother was away. It was interesting to note that a fifth of the ill mothers entered employment during the study year although they had not been working prior to their hospitalization or visit to the emergency services. Incentives to work were given as the need for more family income or the necessity of getting away from household routines and child-care tasks.

The limitations of the person providing child-care were evaluated at the beginning and end of the study year by determining the time available for child-care, the health of the caretaker, the adequacy of the caretaker, and the willingness of the caretaker. The caretakers in the first two studies were mostly fathers or substitute persons while in Study III the ill mothers were in the home and were the caretakers; thus some differences in the adequacy factors existed. For example in Study III with ill mothers a large proportion of families were considered, in the evaluation, to have negative factors in health, adequacy, and willingness while in the two-parent families in Study II there were negatives in the time factor due to the larger number of working fathers who assumed the child-care responsibilities while the mothers were hospitalized. The proportions of both two-parent and one-parent families in the urban study (Study III) with at least two negatives in child-care factors at the beginning of the year were found to be much greater than in the small town and suburban study (Study II). This difference reflected the limitations of the ill mother who was caring for the children in the home as against the substitute caretakers in' Study II. Also in Study III at the end of the year there was little change in the adequacy ratings while in the other studies, when the ill mother had returned home, there was an increase in the health negative but a decrease in the limitation of time for child-care. Thus the adequacy of child-care in the urban families showed little improvement over the study year in spite of efforts by the demonstration workers in the demonstration families. Since so many of the child-care problems had existed for a considerable time, the Study year was undoubtedly too short a time to show marked changes since any such changes would, of necessity, have had to be made by the ill mother or with her consent.

The data in these studies show convincingly that the adequate care of children of all ages is usually seriously at risk when the mother is mentally ill at home or hospitalized and that adequate child-care is less threatened when the fathers rather than the mothers are hospitalized. Children of mentally ill mothers still in the home often presented the most serious problems in the adequacy of child-care.

COMMUNITY RESOURCES

The extent to which these families of mentally ill parents used community agencies was studied by grouping the agencies into seven basic types: public assistance, family agencies, children's agencies, psychiatric resources, correctional programs, medical social service, and public health nursing. Almost half of the families in the three studies were being assisted by at least one of the agencies at the beginning of the studies. One-parent families were using agency help more than two-parent families. The urban families in Study III used agencies more, as did the black families. Less than a fifth of the families were active with two or more agencies at the beginning of the Study year. More two-parent families had had contacts with psychiatric services than one-parent families.

More urban families used agencies providing public assistance, services for children, and psychiatric resources than was true in the small town and suburban families. Public health nursing services were used by more families in Studies I and III than in Study II. However in Study I the public health nurses were primarily involved in the families with tuberculous patients. Thus nursing services were used by more families in the urban study than in the suburban areas.

Larger proportions of demonstration than of control families with ill mothers became known to public assistance and family agencies during the Study year. The increase in the use of family agencies by the demonstration families with ill fathers as well as ill mothers reflects the work of the demonstration workers in seeking these specialized services for families. However some of these referrals to family agencies were for the purpose of securing homemakers. More demonstration than control families maintained contacts with psychiatric agencies during the Study year. This fact indicates the efforts of the demonstration workers in keeping these patients under psychiatric care.

Of interest are the proportions of families for which psychiatric or family services were discontinued during the Study year at a period when families were still involved with the mentally ill parent. In Study III an effort was made to determine from the various agencies the ressons for discontinuing services. The reason given was usually that the families had no further need for service. Psychiatric services frequently reported as reasons lack of cooperation or other difficulties in the patient's use of services. In view of the numerous and, in many families, severe social and health problems in these families as reported by the research interviewers and demonstration workers, it is difficult to agree with the decision of the agencies that there was no further need for services. However one explanation may be that agencies in discontinuing services were relating only to a specific need in the family rather than to the total needs of the family, especially the children. Public assistance agencies usually closed their cases when financial help was no longer needed by the family and similarly family agencies closed cases when homemakers were no longer being used. Frequently when the ill mother returned from the hospital and often needed help and guidance from agencies, agencies tended to discontinue their help. This was true of children's agencies which seemed primarily concerned with meeting the acute or emergency need of the children by providing shelter when the mothers were hospitalized. It was usual that children were returned home, either from agency care or care of relatives, shortly after or often at the same time as the ill mother returned home from the hospital.

The fact that half of the ill mothers in Study III were readmitted to the mental hospital during the Study year may well be related to the fact that they prematurely assumed household and child-care responsibilities which were forced upon them when the resources within the family and in the community folded up. The need for a more gradual plan for assuming responsibilities is obvious and merits community planning in order to make the posthospital course for these ill mothers one of planned rehabilitation as well as to lessen the frequency of readmissions to mental hospitals. The tendency of agencies in general to discontinue treatment regardless of the presence of underlying family problems indicates the present emphasis on short-time services to meet an acute situation with little effort placed on continuing, supportive help to families with mental illness as they struggle to manage in spite of problems with which they need help.

In Study III there was a difference in the agencies' awareness of problems in the demonstration families as contrasted with the control families. This reflects the concern of the demonstration workers that the total problems in a family should be recognized and treated and insofar as possible some preventive services provided. In the demonstration cases some attempt was made by the agencies to deal with more of the problems.

Public assistance, psychiatric, and public health nursing agencies were generally unaware of the problems relating to children and focused their attention mainly on the parents, especially the ill parent. This was also true of problems in marital relations and housing. The number of families known to other types of agencies were too few in number to draw any conclusion but the general impression from the study is that these were also fractionated services and were not concerned with the family's problems as a whole. When agencies were asked by the study staff to identify difficulties in providing services during the study year, the replies from public assistance, family, children, psychiatric, and public health nursing services indicated that there were no difficulties in providing services in over half of the families known to these agencies. These replies probably reflected the limited roles the agencies assumed in their practice even though they might have been aware of more extensive problems. Had they assumed the role as being involved with the range of family and children's problems either by working on these problems themselves or by referral to appropriate agencies, they would have provided more follow-up, more aggressive referrals, and more coordination between their work with the family and the work of other agencies. Furthermore, continuity in services would probably have resulted. It was apparent that when several agencies were working with the family at the same time there was little sharing of knowledge or joint planning about the needs of families.

The reluctance of families to turn to social and health agencies, whether for financial or other reasons, was common; yet, in spite of the limitations in agency roles, most of the demonstration and control families, when asked, reported that agencies had been helpful. Thus, when families had the opportunity to utilize agency services the services appeared to the families to be effective. The problem, therefore, was the lack of availability of services to these families and the limited scope of their programs.

EFFORTS TO ASSIST

The major purposes in the demonstrations in Studies II and III were to determine the extent and severity of problems in a group of families of mentally ill patients to provide, either directly or through referral to appropriate resources, the services needed to lessen or prevent the problems expecially as they related to children, and to find an effective way of assisting families experiencing the impact of mental illness of a parent. There were differences in the organization of the demonstrations in the two studies.

Study II

In Study II community agencies in each of two small cities organized themselves into a committee to receive referrals of families with parents in a state hospital, to assign each family to an agency for continuing services throughout the study year, to follow through with the agencies to ensure adequacy and continuity of care, and to provide the leadership for the project. In one of the demonstration cities a family agency was the pivot agency to coordinate the services, while in the other city it was a mental health center.

Working agreements were drawn up between a state hospital from which the study sample was secured and the social agencies in the demonstration communities. Forms to be filled out by the admitting office which would identify patients with children at home under 18 years were developed by the study staff. The data from these forms proved useful to the hospital staff and was essential in casefinding which led to enlisting the services of agencies in the demonstration communities. The agencies agreed to reach out to offer help to these families in planning for child-care, to assess the physical, social, and emotional problems of the children in these families, and to provide necessary services throughout the study year.

Guidelines, classifying family problems and children's needs to be used for agency evaluations of problems, were developed by the project staff and distributed to agencies for their use. The guidelines also suggested possible ways in which community help might be provided. Three major problem areas of particular significance in child-care were housing, income, and caretakers.

Of the forty-eight demonstration families, thirty-nine families accepted the services of the agencies. The other nine families had refused agency help from the time of the first research interview but agreed to continue with the two subsequent research interviews. Refusals seemed to occur in families of relatively high socioeconomic level, in those related to town officials, and in two instances in families who did not want to reveal embarrassing marital or personal problems.

In the thirty-nine families known to demonstration workers, financial problems were found in 61%, housing difficulties in 32%, and caretaker problems in 52%. In nearly all instances agencies attempted to help families with these problems.

The demonstration showed that the agencies had been able in most instances to make an immediate home visit after referral and that the families welcomed the interest of the agency. However because of the pressures of their regular responsibilities to the community, they were in most instances unable to maintain continuity of service throughout the study year as had been requested.

Because these demonstration families had not themselves asked for agency help, new techniques of reaching-out to offer services to families in their homes were required. Also because of the emphasis on early identification of problems and, wherever possible of preventing problems by anticipating what might happen if certain steps were not taken, new ways of thinking and relating to families varied somewhat from the agencies' usual approach with families who, themselves, asked for help in relation to a recognized problem.

This demonstration also emphasized the need of securing information as to which patients had children at home at the time parents are admitted to state hospitals, and the need to see that these families are, at the time of admission, referred to appropriate social agencies for help in planning for care of their children, at least during the parent's hospitalization. The demonstration showed that such steps would be not only helpful to families but would also help to relieve patients of their worries about the children at home.

The study found that communication between the hospital and the community was usually focused at the point of discharge of the patient and that during the patient's stay in the hospital it had been very difficult, often impossible, for community agencies to secure any information or advice from the hospital that the agency needed in the work with the family, especially in planning for the care of children. In the study the participation of the hospital social worker in the community committee and his availability to confer with agencies facilitated communication between the hospital and the community and resulted in an important community role for the hospital to play. Joint planning also was furthered by the inclusion of agency representation at patient conferences at the hospital which were concerned largely with after-care planning. Thus consideration both of the hospital's role and of the social worker's role as participants in community planning resulted in effective coordination of services.

Study III

Because of these difficulties in securing continuous reaching-out service, Study III was designed to include, on the Study staff, its own demonstration workers who were freed from community pressures to give service to other families. These demonstration workers were responsible for providing social services to the thirty-five demonstration families either directly or through referral to appropriate agencies. The demonstration workers retained interest in the family even when they were known to other agencies in order to ensure comprehensive and continuous service throughout the study year. Because of this the data in Study III is more complete than that in Study II.

Difficulties in family functioning was rated from the demonstration records in relation to twenty problem areas; five related to the ill mother, three to the father, three to the family as a whole, two to the environment, and seven to one or more children in the family. Problems were identified at the beginning and end of the demonstration year. Many of the difficulties were chronic in nature. The most frequent problem areas noted were the mother's physical health, the mother's mental or emotional condition, the mother as a caretaker of children, the marital situation, relations with relatives, leisure time recreation problems, housing and neighborhood limitations, finances, and the children's health. Other problem areas of children less frequently noted were difficulties in school, overt behavioral problems, and those of a psychoneurotic nature. One- and two-parent families in general had similar proportions of these problems except that in one-parent families marital problems were less while those of the mother as a homemaker and those related to her employment were greater.

There was, surprisingly, a smaller proportion of children with neurotic type problems in one-parent families as compared to two-parent families but there was a larger proportion with overt behavioral difficulties in one-parent families. These differences existed in all age groups.

Physical problems reported by the demonstration records were predominant in children of all ages. In the teenage group problems involving behavior and peer relationships were higher. School problems appeared throughout all age groups. Except for a larger proportion of girls than boys aged 6-12 years with sibling problems, the incidence of problems was about the same for both sexes. Problems of physical health, especially the need for dental care and health supervision, were predominant in children of all ages.

The demonstration staff, in their services to families, were involved with problems relating to the ill mother, the father, the family as a whole, and the environment in most families in which there were problems in these areas. However, they were less frequently and less intensively involved with the specific difficulties of children. This was due to the severity of the mother's own problems, to her frequent defensiveness about the worker's relationship with the children, and to the need to work with and through the ill mother before anything could be accomplished directly with the children. Supportive casework was constantly used with these ill mothers, supplemented as the year went on by various forms of guidance and environmental manipulation.

During the year the demonstration staff worked most often with public assistance departments, medical and psychiatric hospitals and clinics, and a group of specialized agencies. The mean number of resources with which the demonstration worker was in communication was six per family, although in some instances there were as many as fourteen. Contacts with psychiatric resources and public assistance were usually for coordination of services; those with family agencies for referral and those with public health nursing for information.

Improvement during the year in relation to individual problem areas was most frequently in the mother's mental health, her role in the care of her children, the father's employment, leisure-recreation, housing, and the children's physical health. The effectiveness of the demonstration work was seen most strongly in the areas of the children's health and of leisure-recreation. Somewhat less effective were the demonstration's efforts in relation to the mother's physical health, her caretaking role, the family's relationship with relatives, finances, and the neurotic and overt behavioral difficulties of children.

The effectiveness of agencies' services was judged in relation to four factors: agency policy, agency practice, family motivation, and continuity of services during the year. Effectiveness of medical and psychiatric practice included such factors as interest shown in the medical or psychiatric problems of the patient and family, follow-up of the pediatrician's recommendations, cooperation with the family and the demonstration, and the organization of services, rather than the actual medical competence of the individual physician or psychiatrist. By far the largest number of families received ineffective services, when judged by those criteria, from psychiatric hospitals and clinics. About a quarter received ineffective service from medical agencies and from public assistance. In relation to other factors—inadequate policies, practice, family "not motivated," and service not continuous—the psychiatric resources again had the highest proportion of ineffective services.

After the end of the Study year, agencies to which the demonstration staff had referred families were requested to report the status of the case. Of the thirteen families referred to agencies it was found that five cases had been closed within 4 to 6 months after referral, another case within 6 weeks, and in another no action had ever been taken by the agency. The remaining six cases were still considered active by the agencies 8 to 15 months after the demonstration year had ended but regular contacts were about to be closed. These thirteen families were referred by the demonstration workers to the agencies because of the serious and complicated problems that had existed in these families for some time. In most of these cases several agencies had been active with the families over the years as crises arose but the services had been mostly time-limited and fractionated. It was the hope and expectation of the demonstration worker that the agency's acceptance of the referral meant that the agency would make a real effort to assist the family with its problems; this would require continuous service for longer than a few weeks or months. The demonstration workers had given these families intensive casework services for a year. The progress was slow but in most cases apparent. In referring these families they made it clear that services would be needed for a long time if much progress was to be reached but that services were essential in order to protect children, if possible, from the results of longer exposure to serious problems existing in these families. The inability of agencies to focus on the total needs of families or to provide continuity of services suggests that in this urban area the agencies are not equipped to meet the needs of children and families with persistent and recurrent problems of serious impact on the well-being of children.

IMPLICATIONS OF THE STUDY

In order to ensure that families, especially children with mentally ill parents, receive the help they need to protect the children and to provide adequate care for them during the parent's illness, two changes are needed: (1) changes in the points of view about providing services, and (2) a change in the organization of services within the community.

The needed changes in points of view include: (1) the need to expand the understanding of what adequate or comprehensive service is and what is required to provide such service; (2) the need to focus on the problems in the total situation rather than just on the patient as an ill person; (3) the need to assess carefully the hazards to children in leaving them in a family with constant stresses due to the parent's mental illness, and to recognize when these hazards are greater than the hazards to children in care elsewhere; (4) the need to consider placement of children away from their own homes before the children are seriously traumatized by the home situation, (5) the need to recognize that employment of the ill mother outside the home may be an important step in her rehabilitation as well as a way of helping the family to cope with the stresses created by mental illness; (6) the need to rethink the concept that only when a client asks for help can services be effective as contrasted with the agency's reaching out to offer services; (7) the need to consider a change in the focus and priorities of health and social services so as to include emphases on preventive measures as well as curative services; (8) the need to emphasize the effectiveness of providing external, supportive services as well as treatment of the psychological problems by the use of environmental manipulation and other positive experiences for patients and their families in an effort to build family strengths; (9) the need to realize that, in families with mentally ill parents, problems have usually existed for a period of time and are so pervasive within the family effecting all members that time is needed to help families with these multiple problems, not just assistance during the period of crises; and (10) the need to change agencies' attitudes toward coordination and collaboration with all other agencies attempting to help a family at the same time.

In order to alleviate the serious impact of mental illness on children some essential steps must be taken immediately. These are: (1) the establishment of a policy in each agency that requires each worker to make a fuller assessment of a family's total situation in order to determine the extent and severity of mental illness in a family and its impact on children, and on the basis of this assessment to provide the needed services either through the agency or by referral to other appropriate resources; (2) the development of a procedure in every mental hospital and psychiatric emergency service that would identify at the time the mentally ill parent is admitted those parents with children at home in order that services to these families may be given at the earliest possible time either directly by the social worker in the emergency service or the hospital or by a community agency which has agreed to accept such referrals; (3) the establishment of more day-care facilities for children which would make it possible for many children to be cared for at home during the mother's illness; (4) the development of day centers for parents recuperating from an acute mental illness as a means of helping the parent to adjust to community life; (5) an expansion of home-help and homemaker services to keep families intact when the mother is hospitalized and to assist her when she goes home in order to relieve the pressures on her which frequently create the need for rehospitalization; (6) extension of psychiatric services into the homes of many of these families to provide a clearer picture of the home situation and continuity of psychiatric care; (7) a further assumption of responsibility by the psychiatric emergency service and hospitals to ensure that no parent is sent home without determining what this will mean to the family and without a definite arrangement with the patient for further psychiatric care and social services either by the hospital or by referral to a community agency; and (8) a closer coordination between the psychiatric and social agencies providing care to the family and the schools the children attend in order that the agencies may be more aware of the impact on the children of the parent's mental illness as seen through the child's school experiences and in order that the schools may be drawn into a coordinated plan of service, hopefully through an expansion of the school social work program.

The studies clearly demonstrated the lack of coordination and collaboration among social, health, and educational programs. In order to develop a system that would prevent gaps and duplications in services it might be possible to assign a coordinating role to an agency. When this was tried in one of these studies it was only partially successful because of the pressures already existing on the agencies. The plan, however, merits application. In it a coordinating committee made up of representatives of health, education, and social services would be responsible for planning the coordination of services in order to ensure a program of comprehensive and continuous care for as long as was needed.

A more ideal organizational plan, however, would be the development of community centers that would be equipped to provide, within the center itself, comprehensive health and social services. The center would provide over-all planning, unified services, and continuous evaluation of the effectiveness of the program. Thus, the family would have one place to go for help with its health and social problems and would see the center as the place to turn to as soon as needs arise rather than delaying until the problems are acute or so chronic that services are ineffective.

Only by some such method of providing comprehensive care to families of mentally ill parents will the incidence and severity of the problems created for children be identified, adequate services provided, and the serious impact lessened. Without such help children will be exposed to the disturbing and disruptive effects of parental mental illness which will contribute to their own emotional problems and may be the foundation of mental illness in the future.

References

Ainsworth; Andry; Harlow; Lebovici; Mead; Prugh; and Wootton. The Effects of Maternal Deprivation: A Review of Findings and Controversy in the Context of Research Strategy. *World Health Organization Public Health Papers*, 1962, **14**, 97-165.

Albert, R. S. Stages of Breakdown in the Relationships and Dynamics Between the Mental Patient and His Family. *American Medical Association Archives of General Psychiatry*, December 1960, **3**, 682-690.

Andry, R. G. *Delinquency and Parental Pathology; A Study in Forensic and Clinical Psychology.* London: Methuen & Co., Ltd., 1960.

Aubry, J. *La Carence de Soins Maternels.* Centre Internat. de l'enfance, Paris: Presses Universitaires de France, 1955.

Bakwin, H. Loneliness in Infants. *American Journal of Diseases of Children*, January 1942, **63**, 30-40.

Bakwin, H. Emotional Deprivation in Infants. *Journal of Pediatrics*, October 1949, **35**, 512-521.

Bellak, L. A General Hospital as a Focus of Community Psychiatry. A Trouble Shooting Clinic Combines Important Functions as a Part of Hospital's Emergency Service. *Journal of the American Medical Association*, December 1960, **174**, 2214-2217.

Bergman, A. B., & Haggerty, R. J. The Emergency Clinic. A Study of Its Role in a Teaching Hospital. *American Journal of Diseases of Children*, July 1962, **104**, 36-44.

Boardman, H. E. Who Insures the Child's Right to Health. *The Neglected Battered-Child Syndrome. Role Reversal in Patients.* Publication G. New York: Child Welfare League of America, Inc., July 1963.

Bowlby, J. Maternal Care and Mental Health. *Bulletin of World Health Organization*, 1951, **3**, 355-533.

Brenneman, J. The Infant Ward. *American Journal of Diseases of Children*, March 1932, **43**, 577-584.

Buckle, D., & Lebovici, S. The Child in the Family. *World Health Organization Public Health Papers*, 1965, **28**, 34-40.

Buell, B. et al. *Community Planning for Human Services.* New York: Columbia University Press, 1952.

Burlingham, D., & Freud, A. *Young Children in Wartime; A Year's Work in a Residential War Nursery.* London: G. Allen & Unwin, Ltd., 1942.

Burlingham, D., & Freud, A. *Infants Without Families; The Case For and Against Residential Nurseries.* London: G. Allen & Unwin, Ltd., 1943.

Chapin, D. A Plea for Accurate Statistics in Infants' Institutions Transactions. *American Journal of Diseases of Children,* 1915, 27, 180-185.

Clausen, J. A., & Yarrow, M. R. (Eds.). The Impact of Mental Illness on the Family. *Journal of Social Issues,* 1955, 11, 3.

Coleman, J. V., A Community Project in Behalf of the Hospitalized Mentally Ill Patient: The Cooperative Care Project. *American Journal of Psychiatry,* July 1967, 124, 76-79.

Coleman, J. V., & Errera, P. The General Hospital Emergency Room and Its Psychiatric Problems. *American Journal of Public Health,* August 1963, 53, 1294-1301.

Coleman, M. D., & Zwerling, I. The Psychiatric Emergency Clinic: A Flexible Way of Meeting Community Mental Health Needs. *American Journal of Psychiatry,* May 1959, 115, 980-984.

Cowie, V. The Incidence of Neurosis in the Children of Psychotics. *Acta Psychiatrica Scandinaca,* 1961, 37, 37-87.

Crocetti, G. M., & Lemkau, P. V. Public Opinion of Psychiatric Home Care in an Urban Area. *American Journal of Public Health,* March 1963, 53, 409-417.

Deane, W. N. The Handling of Pathological and Institutionally Induced Psychotic Remnants in Socially Recovered Schizophrenic Patients. *Mental Hygiene,* July 1963, 47, 477-482.

Detre, T. P., Kessler, D. R., & Jarecki, H. G. The Role of the General Hospital in Modern Community Psychiatry. *American Journal of Orthopsychiatry,* July 1963, 33, 690-700.

Division of Public Health Methods, U.S. Department of Health, Education, and Welfare. *Homemaker Services in the United States, 1958. Twelve Statements Describing Different Types of Homemaker Services.* Public Health Services Publication 645. Washington: U.S. Government Printing Office, 1958.

Doniger, C. R. Children Whose Mothers Are in a Mental Hospital. *Journal of Child Psychology and Psychiatry and Allied Disciplines,* July-December, 1962, 3, 165-173.

Freeman, H., & Farndale, J. (Eds.). *Trends in the Mental Health Services; A Symposium of Original and Reprinted Papers.* London: Pergamon Press, Ltd., 1963.

Freeman, H. E., & Simmons, O. G. Treatment Experiences of Mental Patients and Their Families. *American Journal of Public Health,* September 1961, 51, 1266-1273.

Freeman, H. E.. *The Mental Patient Comes Home.* New York: John Wiley & Sons, Inc., 1963.

Freund, W. VIII. Uber den "Hospitalismus" der Sauglinge Ergebnisse der Inneren. *Medizin und Kinderheilkunde,* 1910, 6, 333-368.

Friedman, T. T., Rolfe, P., & Perry, S. E. Home Treatment of Psychiatric Patients. *American Journal of Psychiatry,* March 1960, 116, 807-809.

Hill, R. et al. *Families Under Stress; Adjustment to the Crises of War Separation and Reunion.* New York: Harper & Row, 1949.

Hill, R. C. Social Stresses on the Family. 1. Generic Features of Families Under Stress. *Social Casework,* February-March 1958, 39, 139-150.

Hoenig, J., & Hamilton, M. W. Extramural Care of Psychiatric Patients. *Lancet,* 19 June 1965, 1, 1322-1325.

Hollingshead, A. G., & Redlich, F. C. *Social Class and Mental Illness*: A Community Study, New York: John Wiley & Sons, Inc., 1958.

Hollis, F. *Casework, A Psychosocial Therapy.* New York: Random House, 1964.

Ingham, H. V. Statistical Study of Family Relationships in Psychoneurosis. *American Journal of Psychiatry,* August 1949, 106, 91-98.

Joint Commission on Mental Illness and Health. *Action for Mental Health: Final Report of the Joint Commission on Mental Illness and Health, 1961.* New York: Basic Books, Inc., 1961.

Koos, E. L. *Families in Trouble.* Monograph, New York: Kings Crown Press, 1946.

Lemkau, P. V., & Crocetti, G. The Amsterdam Municipal Psychiatric Service: A Psychiatric-Sociological Review. *American Journal of Psychiatry,* March 1961, 117, 779-783.

Margolis, P. M. Stabilizing the Family Through Homemaker Service. *Social Casework,* October 1957, 38, 412-416.

McClellan, S. G., & Pugh, T. F. Childhood Development Following Maternal Mental Illness. Paper presented at the 90th Annual Meeting, American Public Health Association, Miami, Florida, October 16, 1962. (Mimeographed.)

McNair, F. E., & Elmore, E. A Sustaining Service for Discharged Mental Hospital Patients. *Canadian Medical Association Journal,* 7 October 1961, 85, 810 811.

Method and Process in Social Casework. Family Service Association of America, 1958.

Miller, A. A Report on Psychiatric Emergencies. *Canadian Hospitals,* December 1959, 36, 36-37.

Pennell, M. Y., & Smith, L. M. Characteristics of Families Served by Homemakers. *American Journal of Public Health,* November 1959, 49, 1467-1474.

Radinsky, E. K. Children of Discharged Mental Hospital Patients. *Children,* May-June 1961, 8, 88-92.

Ribble, M. A. *Rights of Infants; Early Psychological Needs and Their Satisfaction.* 22nd ed. New York: Columbia University Press, 1943.

Ross Laboratories. Protecting Children of the Mentally Ill. *Currents in Public Health*, June 1965, 5, 1.

Skudder, P. A., McCarrol, J. R. & Wade, P. A. Hospital Emergency Facilities and Services, A Survey. *Bulletin of American College of Surgeons*, March-April 1961, 46, 44-50.

Smith, L. H. New Horizons in Psychiatric Hospitalization. The Psychiatric Revolution. *Journal of the American Medical Association,* 12 November 1960, 174, 1382-1385.

Sobel, D. E. Children of Schizophrenic Patients: Preliminary Observations on Early Development. *American Journal of Psychiatry*, December 1961, 118, 512-517.

Spiegel, J. P., & Bell, N. W. The Family of the Psychiatric Patient *American Handbook of Psychiatry*, New York: Basic Books, Inc., 1959, I, 114-149.

Spitz, R. A. Hospitalism. An Inquiry into the Genesis of Psychiatric Conditions in Early Childhood. *The Psychoanalytic Study of the Child*, New York: International Universities Press, 1945, I, 53-74.

Spitz, R. A., & Wolf, L. M. Anaclitic Depression. An Inquiry into the Genesis of Psychiatric Conditions in Early Childhood. *The Psychoanalytic Study of the Child*, New York: International Universities Press, 1946, II, 313-342.

Stewart, W. H., Pennell, M. Y., & Smith, L. M. *Homemaker Services in the United States, 1958*. A Nationwide Study. Public Health Service Publication 644. Washington: U.S. Government Printing Office, 1958.

Strickler, M., Bassin, E. G., Malbin, V., et al. The Community-Based Walk-In Center: A New Resource for Groups Underrepresented in Outpatient Treatment Facilities. *American Journal of Public Health*, March 1965, 55, 377-384.

Sussex, J. N. Factors Influencing the Emotional Impact on Children of an Acutely Psychotic Mother in the Home. *Southern Medical Journal,* November 1963, 56, 1245-1249.

Sussex, J. N., Gassman, F., & Raffel, S. C. Adjustment of Children with Psychotic Mothers in the Home. *American Journal of Orthopsychiatry*, October 1963, 33, 849-854.

Treudley, M. B. Mental Illness and Family Routines. *Mental Hygiene*, April 1946, 30, 235-249.

Ungerleider, J. T. The Psychiatric Emergency. Analysis of Six Months; Experience of a University Hospital's Consultation Service. *American Medical Association Archives of General Psychiatry*, December 1960, 3, 593-601.

Weinerman, E. R., & Edwards, H. R. "Triage" System Shows Promise in Management of Emergency Department Load. *Hospitals, Journal of American Hospital Association,* 16 November 1964, 38, 55-62.

Weinerman, E. R., Ratner, R. S., Robbins, A., & Lavenhar, M. A. Yale Studies in Ambulatory Medical Care. V. Determinants of Use of Hospital Emergency Services. *American Journal of Public Health*, July 1966, 56, 1037-1056.

Younghusband, E. *Social Work and Social Change.* New York, Council on Social Work Education, 1969.

Index

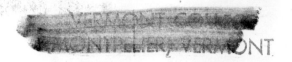
DATE DUE

OCT 1 - '75		
OCT 3 '75		
OCT 2 3 '75		
FEB 23 '77		
APR 1 5 '77		
NOV 7 '77		
NOV 1 7 '77		
AP 2 4 '78		
OCT 3 0 1979		
NOV 1 4 1979		
APR 3 1981		
NOV 9 1981		
		PRINTED IN U.S.A.

GAYLORD